THE ESSENCE OF YOGA

THE ESSENCE OF YOGA

Reflections on the *Yoga Sūtras* of Patañjali

BERNARD BOUANCHAUD

Translated from the French
by Rosemary Desneux

Foreword by
T.K.V. Desikachar

RUDRA PRESS
Portland, Oregon

Rudra Press, PO Box 13390, Portland, Oregon 97213
Telephone: 503-235-0175
Telefax: 503-235-0909

Originally published in French by Éditions Ägamât, 17 Rue Élisée-Reclus, 91120 Palaiseau, France, 1995, ISBN 2-911166-02-7

Cover and text design by Bill Stanton
Cover photograph by Bob Waldman
Typography by William H. Brunson, Typography Services

Library of Congress Cataloging-in-Publication Data

Bouanchaud, Bernard.
[Miroir. English]
The essence of Yoga : reflections on the Yoga sutras of Patañjali / Bernard Bounchaud ; translated from the French by Rosemary Desneux ; foreword by T.K.V. Desikachar.
cm.
Includes bibliographical references.
ISBN 0-915801-69-8 (alk. paper)
1. Patañjali. Yogasutra. 2. Yoga. I. Desneux, Rosemary. II. Title
B132.Y6B66813 97-6643
181′.452—dc21 CIP

01 00 99 98 97 10 9 8 7 6 5 4 3 2 1

To my wife
Johanna Maria Tuinenburg

You can plumb the depths of a well, but the depths of the mind are unfathomable.

—Indian proverb

CONTENTS

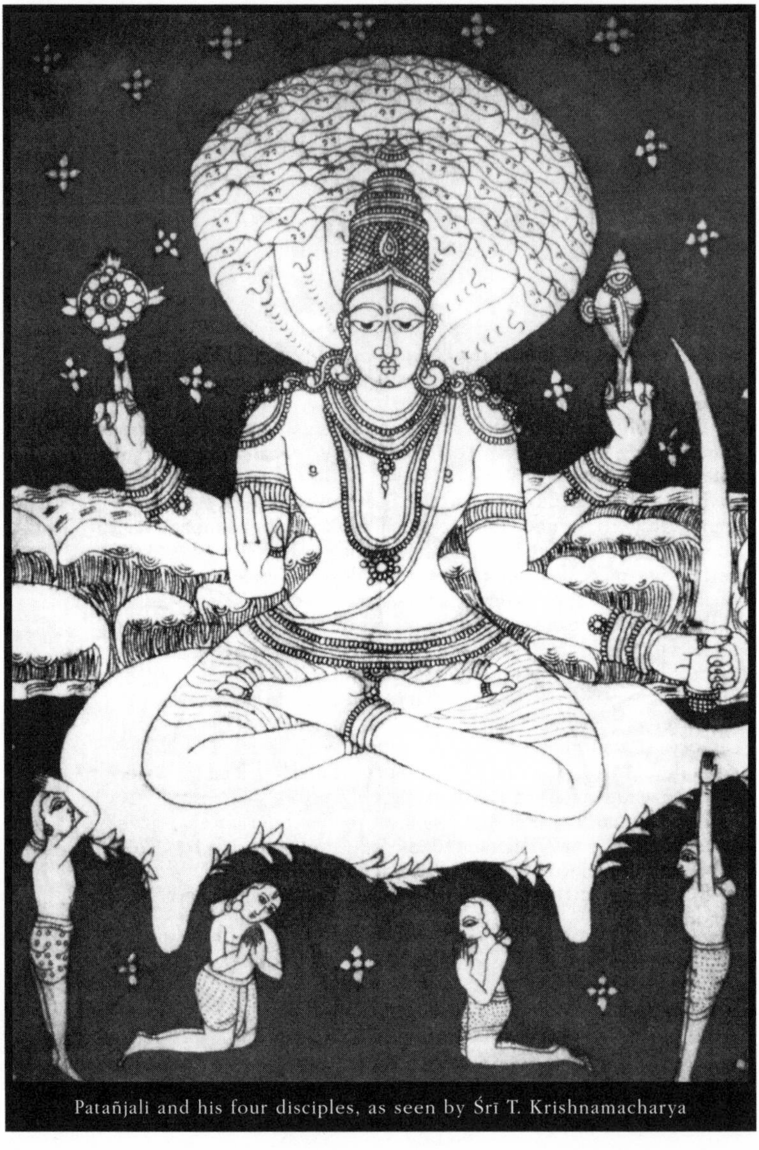

Patañjali and his four disciples, as seen by Śrī T. Krishnamacharya

FOREWORD

Our great traditions, whose origins are so mysterious, have never been obscured by time. This is why they are called eternal teachings.

They were the visions of great seers whose perceptions transcended time and space. No wonder they continue to inspire us. The *Yoga Sūtras* of Patañjali are one of these great traditions. One finds in them a profoundly rich view of what this world is all about and how we should relate to it. In a way, the *sūtras* reveal our own true nature. That is why they are called *yoga-darśanam*—(*darśanam* means vision).

Presented in such brevity, they would remain out of reach if not for the great masters who experienced the message and transmitted it to their disciples. My father, T. Krishnamacharya, was one such master. To bring to light his teaching, which always respected the present moment, is a great task. Having followed the labor of Bernard, I know he has accomplished this enormous task in a way that a reader can pursue with the greatest benefit.

Needless to add, the aspirant can then look for a master with whom to delve deeply into this study and discover one's self. If this is achieved, then the hard work of Bernard is well rewarded.

T.K.V. Desikachar

INTRODUCTION

Long before we detect this precious gem, sheltered from our gaze, the pearl forms slowly in the heart of an oyster. To discover this jewel in the depths and bring it to the surface, a diver may need to train and prepare for years.

So it is with the secret wealth we can find in this ancient text on yoga. It reveals deep riches for those who, through discipline and patience, plumb the depths of the self for the light of universal wisdom. The *Yoga Sūtras* of Patañjali constitute an authoritative treatise on yoga as a discipline of mind, body, and spirit, a way of wisdom born in India. Its origins are as invisible and mysterious as those of a spring to which we are drawn to quench our thirst for knowledge.

Yoga is one of the six classical philosophical systems, or *darśanam,* of India. One meaning of *darśanam* is mirror, and as such it is a means of revealing the self. India's sacred texts assert that God was the first yogi; the word *Patañjali* signifies that with hands harmoniously curved and joined, we cup them together to catch yoga's wisdom. The *Yoga Sūtras* of Patañjali will assist us in this. Recognized by all branches of yoga, its inspiration comes from the *Vedas,* a collection of very ancients texts that are the foundation of the Hindu spiritual tradition. However, the origins of yoga's wisdom are not what really concerns us; rather, we wish to study it seriously and reap its benefits.

The origin of the *Yoga Sūtras* lies between the fourth century BCE and the fourth century CE. Though little is know of the author, Patañjali, legend tells us the origin of the text: The human race in its distress prayed to God for enlightenment. God sent a sage who composed three treatises in response to human difficulties:

- One, on medicine, *Caraka Saṃhitá,* taught us the art of healing.
- Another, on grammar, *Mahābhāṣyam,* taught us the art of communication.
- The third, on yoga, taught us the way to a peaceful mind and spiritual growth.

The *Yoga Sūtras* were handed down through oral tradition. Under the master's supervision, a disciple learned the 195 sutras (196 in some schools) by heart. The brevity and simplicity of these sutras, or aphorisms, is a hallmark of oral tradition that allowed perfect memo-

nd pronunciation. This ensured the integrity of the text own from generation to generation; it also embodied the spirit of yoga and the need for direct experience of it. Only when the disciple mastered memorization and pronunciation could he begin to question his understanding.

These aphorisms provide deep, universal insight into the essential psychological, philosophical, and metaphysical questions we pose. They do not resolve questions concerning the creation and origin of the world, but instead address our understanding of the more immediate preoccupations of our essential being: the causes of suffering and how to reduce them.

The four chapters of sutras progressively weave together as a harmonious whole, yet each chapter also presents a coherent teaching in itself. According to Śrī T. Krishnamacharya,* Patajali conceived each chapter in turn with one of his four chief disciples in mind: Mastakāñjali, Kṛtāñjali, Baddhāñjali, and Pūrṇañjali.

These four chapters correspond to various personal inclinations related to temperament, socio-professional situations, and so on, and this is reflected in the chapter titles.

Chapter I	Contemplation
Chapter II	Method
Chapter III	Exceptional Faculties
Chapter IV	Serenity

When beginning study of the sutras, the student uses a personal approach based on experience rather than simply following the chronological order of the chapters. Thus, somebody who is actively employed might start with Chapter II, which discusses day to day difficulties, before studying Chapter I, which presents contemplation as one of the highest aims of yoga. Chapters III and IV examine the higher capacities we can develop through yoga and the highest goal attainable by a human being.

As interest in yoga increases in the West, one danger that arises is oversimplification—reducing yoga to a purely physical discipline. Another problem is seeing yoga as a purely esoteric quest, particularly due to the difficulty of reading original texts on yoga. In this light, Patañjali's treatise, which is extremely concise, is meant to be commented on and explained during oral exchanges. Its teaching is uniquely adapted to each personality and its semantic richness

*Śrī Krishnamacharya was an Indian yogi who died at the age of 100 in Madras in 1988. His life was dedicated to restoring the universal value of the *Yoga Sūtras* to yoga. He had many famous disciples, including his own son, Śrī T.K.V. Desikachar.

allows for multidimensional levels of interpretation, but this also can render understanding difficult, especially to nonspecialists.

The work presented here attempts to meld precise and simple commentary with personal study, supplying explanations and themes for reflection for each aphorism. This will be most fruitful for readers willing to question themselves. A first reading can open the way; however only discussions in private with an experienced guide can lead to real liberation.

The goal of this book is to facilitate the search for inner balance and personal growth through a better knowledge of yourself and your real potential. The emphasis is on using the text to free yourself from past conditioning through self-discovery in the mirror of yoga, which throws a new light on everything. To progress, the individual approach must be daily, long-term, and ever-renewed. Benefits may not be recognized immediately; they may come only after several months, perhaps even years, of practice, study, and persevering reflection. But what joy when the veil is torn from our eyes and we discover real inner freedom! May each reader find in their endeavor the strength and determination to continue on the road to self-liberation.

This work, therefore, is not a comparative study of the *Yoga Sūtras,* but reflection based on oral transmission.* Patañjali's text is set out aphorism by aphorism, with each including:

- a translation, rarely literal, that aims at transmitting the aphorism's essential message in a form usable by Westerners today
- themes for personal reflection
- commentary that provides a foundation for reflection
- the original sanskrit text
- the same text with caesuras: we have retained declensions in order to present, in many cases, a literal translation with prepositions and other elements that elucidate the word function in the aphorism
- word-by-word translation

Palaiseau, France
17 May 1995

*The written text is taken from the *Yoga Sūtras Workbook,* published in Madras by the Krishnamacharya Yoga Mandiram.

SANSKRIT TRANSLITERATION AND PRONUNCIATION

The most widely used script in India for Sanskrit is the *devangārī.*

The table on the next page shows:

- the Sanskrit alphabet in *devanāgarī* script
- transliteration of each letter, with classical diacritics. These are placed under the letter in *devanāgarī.*

Pronunciation very often differs from English:

- *u* = ou (*guru* = gourou, as in English through)
- *ṛ* = ri, rolled r (*vṛtti* = *vritti*)
- *i, u, ṛ, ḷ,* short vowels
- *ī, ū, ṛ, e, ai, au,* long vowels
- *ṃ* (*anusvāra*) nasalization of the preceding vowel
- *ḥ* (visarga) muted expiration
- *e* = (veda = veida as in veil)
- *kh, gh, ch, jh, h, h, th, dh, ph, bh, h* = clearly audible aspiration
- *g* = g hard (*gītā* = guita as in guitar)
- *c* = tch (*cakra* = tchakra)
- *j* = dj (*japa* = djapa as in judge)
- *ṭ, ṭh, ḍ, ḍh* = tip of the tongue turned upwards
- *n* = is pronounced (*yogin* = yoguinn as in inn)
- *ś*= German ch ich (Śiva = shiva, English shin)
- *ṣ*= ch (purua = pourousha)
- *s* = ss (āsana = āssana as in ass

अ	आ	इ	ई	उ	ऊ	ऋ	ॠ	ळ	ए	ऐ	ओ	औ	अं	अः
a	ā	i	ī	u	ū	ṛ	ṝ	ḷ	e	ai	o	au	ṃ	ḥ

क्	ख्	ग्	घ्	ङ्
k	kh	g	gh	ṅ
च्	छ्	ज्	झ्	ञ्
c	ch	j	jh	ñ
ट्	ठ्	ड्	ढ्	ण्
ṭ	ṭh	ḍ	ḍh	ṅ
त्	थ्	द्	ध्	न्
t	th	d	dh	n
प्	फ्	ब्	भ्	म्
p	ph	b	bh	m
य्	र्	ल्	व्	
y	r	l	v	
श्	ष्	स्		
ś	ṣ	s		
ह	क्ष	ज्ञ		
h	kṣa	jña		

APHORISMS ON YOGA

Since each aphorism is understood only in relation to the others, and its meaning reveals itself slowly, little by little, are my determination and patience up to this task?

To what extent does our interaction with others contribute to self-discovery? Do my personal relationships play a role?

The word *sūtra* is defined as follows:

alpakṣaram asandigdhaṃ saravat viṣvatomukham
aṣtobham anavadyam ca sūtram sūtravido viduḥ

"Spare in its letters, unequivocal, constant, universal, without digressions and pertinently worded, that is what those acquainted with these aphorisms often say about them."

Sūtra is a generic term for treatises written in the form of aphorisms. It also means rope, cord, string, thread (the sacred thread that brahmins, in particular, wear), belt, or a rule expressed briefly in aphorisms. Each aphorism is linked to all the others by this thread. Each can only be understood in relation to each of the others and to the *Yoga Sūtras* as a whole.

The word *yoga* has numerous meanings, of which the first is that of binding or union. It can also designate a vehicle, the use of equipment, a means, a method, a trick, an aptitude, taking possession of, an astronomical conjunction, or an arithmetical addition. Here, its meaning it threefold:

- one of the six classical systems of Indian thought
- a particular state of concentration
- the means, as a whole, leading up to this state

Yoga Sūtras

Yoga: yoga, one of the six traditional systems of thought that refer back to the *Vedas:* (from *yuj*: harness together, hitch up). *Sūtra*: treatise composed of aphorisms; aphorism, cord, thread.

COMPLETE LIST OF SUTRAS

I.1 Now is set forth authoritative teaching on yoga.

I.2 Yoga is the ability to direct and focus mental activity.

I.3 With the attainment of focused mind, the inner being establishes itself in all its reality.

I.4 Otherwise, we identify with the activities of the mind.

I.5 Mental activities are of five kinds, whether they produce suffering or not.

I.6 The five mental activities are: understanding, error, imagination, deep sleep, and memory.

I.7 Understanding arises from sensory perception, inference, and faithful testimony.

I.8 Error is incorrect knowledge based on misinterpretation of reality.

I.9 Imagination is knowledge based on words that have no real, corresponding object.

I.10 Deep sleep is a state of unconscious mental activity in which the four other mental activities are eclipsed.

I.11 Memory retains living experience.

I.12 Control over the mind's fluctuations comes from persevering practice and nonattachment.

I.13 Persevering practice is the effort to attain and maintain the state of mental peace.

I.14 Such a practice is firmly established only if one engages in it seriously and respectfully over a long and uninterrupted period.

I.15 Nonattachment is the mastery of desire for perceived external objects, as well as for internal spiritual objects, heard or revealed.

I.16 At its highest level, nonattachment means having no desire for any of the constituent qualities of nature, because one has become conscious of the spiritual principle.

I.17 Perfect contemplation with full consciousness of the object passes, becoming reflective contemplation, then intuitive, then beatific, and lastly, full consciousness of self in the experience.

I.18 Regular immersion in contemplation without mental fluctuation brings contemplation in which only mental permeation subsists.

I.19 This state is innate for two kinds of predestined beings: those "without a body" and those who are reabsorbed into original matter.

I.20 For the others, faith engenders energy that reinforces the memory, allowing concentration on wisdom.

I.21 For those impelled by intense ardor, the goal is near.

I.22 There still remains a difference based on distinct temperaments: gentle, moderate, and lively.

I.23 Otherwise, the goal is attained by active devotion to God.

I.24 God is a supreme being free from all causes of suffering—from actions, their consequences, and all latency.

I.25 God (vara) is the unequaled source of all knowledge.

I.26 Unsubjected to time, God is the spiritual guide even for the ancients.

I.27 Its expression is the sacred syllable.

I.28 Repeating the sacred syllable and pondering its meaning lead to its understanding.

I.29 It is then that one understands the self and gradually clears inner obstacles.

I.30 The inner obstacles that disperse the mind are sickness, mental inertia, doubt, haste, apathy, intemperance, errors in judgment of oneself, lack of perseverance, and the inability to stay at a level once reached.

I.31 Suffering, depression, physical restlessness, and disturbed breathing accompany mental dispersion.

I.32 The persevering practice of a single principle keeps obstacles at a distance.

I.33 The mind becomes quiet when it cultivates friendliness in the presence of happiness, active compassion in the presence of unhappiness, joy in the presence of virtue, and indifference toward error.

I.34 The mind also attains serenity through prolonged exhalation and holding the breath.

I.35 Objective sensory perception stabilizes and focuses thought.

I.36 Mental stability also stems from serenity linked to luminous lucidity.

I.37 Turning to a being whose mind is released from passions is also calming.

I.38 Mental stability also flows from the consciousness in dream and deep sleep.

I.39 Choosing meditation according to one's affinities also brings mental stability.

I.40 Control of the mind then extends to the infinitely small and the infinitely vast.

I.41 As fluctuations subside, the contemplative mind becomes transparent like a gem, and reflects the object, whether it is that which perceives, the instrument of perception, or the object perceived.

I.42 It then becomes contemplation with a mixed approach, in which representations of the object remain: its name, its essence, and the knowledge one has of it.

I.43 Beyond the mixed approach stage, contemplation manifests the exact nature of the object. Memory is totally purified, as if the mind were stripped of its identity.

I.44 Such contemplation intuitively grasps subtle objects in their reality and beyond.

I.45 Subtlety of the object is limitless, except that it must manifest itself.

I.46 These four contemplative stages comprise contemplation with seed.

I.47 With the mastery of the fourth seed of contemplation, the inner being appears in all clarity and serenity.

I.48 Now the outflowing of supreme knowledge is absolute truth.

I.49 This supreme knowledge grasps the intrinsic nature of the object, which differs from the correct knowledge that tradition and inference bring.

I.50 Mental permeation born of direct knowledge opposes all other mental permeation.

I.51 In passing beyond this last kind of mental permeation, seedless contemplation appears.

II.1 The yoga of action is a way of discipline involving self-reflection based on the sacred texts, and surrendering the fruits of action to a higher force.

II.2 The intent is to gradually attain the state of contemplation and diminish the causes of suffering.

II.3 The causes of suffering are ignorance, consciousness of I (egoism), attachment, repulsion, and fear.

II.4 Ignorance is the source of the other four causes of suffering, whether these are latent, feeble, intermittent, or intense.

II.5 Ignorance is the confusion of the temporary with the permanent, the pure with the impure, anguish with the pleasure of being, and the relative with the absolute.

II.6 Individual ego consciousness of "I" sees mental and physical activity as the source of consciousness.

II.7 Attachment is the consequence of pleasure.

II.8 Aversion is the consequence of displeasure.

II.9 Fear is present even for the sage and develops from its own inherent source.

II.10 Recognizing inherent impulses eliminates the causes of suffering at a subtle level.

II.11 Meditation eliminates mental fluctuations set in motion by erroneous impulses.

II.12 Acts stemming from mental disturbance leave imprints that always show themselves in some form or other, visible or invisible.

II.13 When these causes engender acts, their effects influence existence, time, and the experience of events.

II.14 The three kinds of conditioning produce pleasure if the origin is positive, and torment if it is disturbed.

II.15 The discerning person sees that all is suffering, because of changes due to the passage of time, to worries and conditioning, and to inappropriate manifestations of the constituent qualities of nature.

II.16 Future suffering should be avoided.

II.17 The cause of pain is the union between the inner being who perceives and that which is perceived.

II.18 What is perceived has clarity, movement, and inertia and is made up of the elements and the eleven senses. It can lead to sensory experience and to deliverance.

II.19 The origin and characteristics of things are perceived or not perceived.

II.20 The perceiving entity can only perceive. It uses the mind to experiment, but remains unaltered itself.

II.21 What is perceived exists only to serve as object for the perceiving entity.

II.22 What is perceived no longer exists for the perceiving entity once the intent is fulfilled, but it still exists to serve others.

II.23 The union of that which is perceived and the perceiving entity permits understanding of their respective faculties.

II.24 The cause of this union is ignorance.

II.25 When ignorance vanishes, so does union. Its absence brings serenity.

II.26 Awareness of unequivocal discernment ends confused union.

II.27 The ultimate wisdom that emerges has seven stages.

II.28 Eliminating impurity through continued practice of the eight limbs of yoga brings discernment and clear perception.

II.29 The eight limbs of yoga are: respect toward others, self-restraint, posture, breath control, detaching at will from the senses, concentration, meditation, and contemplation.

II.30 The principles of respect for others include nonviolence, truth, honesty, moderation, and noncovetousness.

II.31 When unaffected by social or geographic considerations, or considerations of time or circumstances, these principles are universal. They are the supreme ideals.

II.32 The five personal principles of positive action are purity, contentment, a disciplined life, study of the sacred texts, and worship of God.

II.33 When harassed by doubt, cultivate the opposite mental attitude.

II.34 Cultivating the opposite mental attitude is realizing that it is our own impatience, greed, anger, or aberration that leads us to think, provoke, and approve conflicting thoughts, such as violence. The intensity of such thoughts may be weak, medium, or strong, but their consequences, ever self-perpetuating, are always suffering and ignorance.

II.35 Around one who is solidly established in nonviolence, hostility disappears.

II.36 For one established in truth, the result fits the action.

II.37 All the jewels appear for one who is firmly set in honesty.

II.38 Vitality appears in one who is firmly set in moderation.

II.39 One who perseveres on the path of noncovetousness gains deep understanding of the meaning of life.

II.40 Purity protects one's body and brings nonphysical relationships with others.

II.41 Then, purity, clarity, and well-being of the spirit come to flower, as well as concentration, mastery of the eleven sense organs, and perception of the inner being.

II.42 Contentment brings supreme happiness.

II.43 By eliminating impurity, a disciplined life brings perfection and mastery to the body and the eleven sense organs.

II.44 Union with the chosen divinity comes from the study of self through the sacred texts.

II.45 Contemplation and its powers are attained through worship of God.

II.46 The posture is firm and soft.

II.47 The posture is attained by pacification through correct effort and contemplating the infinite.

II.48 As a result, one is invulnerable to dualism.

II.49 Once this is reached, breath control is the regulation of inhalation and exhalation.

II.50 The phases of breathing are exhalation, inhalation, and suspension. Observing them in space, time, and number, one is able to render breathing more harmonious in duration and subtlety.

II.51 The fourth type of breath control transcends external or internal domains.

II.52 Then, all that veils clarity of perception is swept away.

II.53 And thought becomes fit for concentration.

II.54 Withdrawal of the senses occurs when the sensory organs, independent of their particular objects, conform to the nature of mind.

II.55 It is then that the senses are perfectly mastered.

III.1 Concentration is focusing the mind on a particular point.

III.2 Meditation is the uninterrupted flow of knowledge on this particular point.

III.3 When the object of meditation alone shines in the mind, as though the mind is emptied of its own form—that is contemplation.

III.4 Perfect mastery is prolonged focus on one object through sustained states of concentration, meditation, and contemplation.

III.5 The light of the highest knowledge comes from acquisition of this perfect mastery.

III.6 This perfect mastery is necessary to the stages that remain.

III.7 The last three limbs of yoga are more internal than the first five.

III.8 These last three limbs must themselves be seen as external compared to contemplation without a seed.

III.9 When after a moment of stability, the mind ceases its fluctuation and remains naturally quiet, it begins its transformation to stability.

III.10 This peaceful flow within the mind is born of its own latent impressions.

III.11 In the transformation to contemplation, distraction vanishes and the mind becomes focused.

III.12 Following contemplation is transformation to one-pointedness, in which one experiences with equanimity both mental peace and the return to a less coherent former state.

III.13 The evolution of fundamental tendencies, of relationship to time, and of situations, all of which intervene in the physical constitution and the organs of perception and action, is thus explained.

III.14 One substratum contains past, present, and future characteristics.

III.15 Different methods produce different changes.

III.16 Knowledge of the past and the future proceeds from the mastery of threefold evolution: fundamental, temporal, and situational.

III.17 Interaction among words, their objects, and one's image or idea engenders confusion. Mastering distinction among them allows understanding of the sounds that creatures make.

III.18 Knowledge about the origins of previous stages appears when we gain insight into our own conditioning.

III.19 Knowing what another is thinking comes from perfect mastery of the mind's contents.

III.20 The origin of another's thought is not grasped, because it cannot be observed.

III.21 Invisibility comes from perfect mastery of physical appearance, which allows one to dissociate the observer's gaze from one's own emanations.

III.22 Perfect mastery of slow and rapid evolution of actions brings knowledge of the time and circumstances of one's own death. This is also known through premonition.

III.23 Perfect mastery of friendship and other qualities confers corresponding power.

III.24 By perfect concentration on the elephant and other models, one gains their corresponding strengths.

III.25 Joining the intelligence of the heart with the overflowing of the mind brings knowledge of the subtle or causal, the hidden or unusual, and the physically and psychologically remote.

III.26 Perfect concentration on the sun bestows knowledge of the universe.

III.27 Perfect concentration on the moon bestows knowledge of star patterns.

III.28 Perfect concentration on the polestar bestows knowledge of the movement of the stars.

III.29 Perfect concentration on the energy center of the navel affords knowledge of the body and its physiology.

III.30 Perfect concentration on the throat frees one from hunger and thirst.

III.31 Perfect concentration on the "tortoise channel" brings stability.

III.32 Perfect concentration on the spiritual light at the top of the head brings visions of realized beings.

III.33 Or else, through intuition, all is known.

III.34 Perfect concentration on the heart reveals the contents of the mind.

III.35 The spiritual entity is independent of pacified consciousness. Confusing them only brings a reflection of the spiritual entity. Perfect concentration on their difference brings recognition of the spiritual entity.

III.36 It is then that the faculties of premonition, clairaudience, subtle touch, clairvoyance, refined taste, and sensitive sense of smell appear.

III.37 These faculties are obstacles in contemplation, but powers in active life.

III.38 Letting go of the structure of personality and refining perception of movement awakens the faculty of influencing another's mind and body.

III.39 With perfect mastery of rising vital energy, one rises above water, mud, and thorns.

III.40 Perfect mastery of the vital energy of assimilation and equilibrium brings radiance.

III.41 Perfect mastery of the relationship between the ear and space brings extraordinary hearing.

III.42 Mastering the relationship between the body and ether, then meditating on the lightness of cotton, brings displacement in space.

III.43 When outside things no longer condition mental activity, the veil over the light of understanding is rent asunder and a state of liberation appears.

III.44 Mastering the material—the real form, the causal structure, concrete possibilities, and value based on the goal—brings mastery of the five elements.

III.45 Perfect mastery of the five elements brings mastery of physical form, physical vigor, and freedom from physical constraint.

III.46 Physical plenitude consists in physical beauty, charm, strength, and being as solid as a diamond.

III.47 Perfect mastery of perception, of the perceived object, of the perceiving entity, of the reference in oneself, and of the intent, brings mastery of the organs of perception, action, and thought.

III.48 Then, instantaneous thought, perception independent of the sense organs, and perfect mastery of origins appear.

III.49 Complete revelation of the difference between the perceiving entity and the mind at peace brings omniscience and omnipotence.

III.50 Spiritual liberation comes when we renounce even omniscience and omnipotence, and when the origin of personal causes of suffering is destroyed.

III.51 When higher creatures invite you, do not give way to wonderment on meeting them, but keep a detached viewpoint when faced with their allure.

III.52 Perfect mastery of the instant and its unfolding brings knowledge born of highly distinctive perception.

III.53 This specific knowledge allows differentiation between two objects otherwise indistinguishable by origin, characteristics, or situation.

III.54 Such is knowledge born of discrimination—it flows spontaneously and pertains to any object, at any level.

III.55 When the purity of the peaceful mind is identical with that of the spiritual entity, that is liberation.

IV.1 Superior faculties originate from birth, the use of consecrated plants, recitation of mantra, ascetic discipline, and contemplation.

IV.2 Positive evolution is the result of one's innermost nature.

IV.3 The causes of evolution do not set nature in motion, but withdraw obstacles, like a gardener opening an irrigation canal.

IV.4 Individual consciousness develops only in contact with another individual consciousness.

IV.5 A single individual consciousness is operative over many others in varied manifestations.

IV.6 Then, that which arises from meditation produces no negative influence over others.

IV.7 The yogi's action is neither black nor white; the action of others is of three kinds.

IV.8 Consequences surely follow these inappropriate tendencies.

IV.9 Despite differences in birth, place, and era, our behavior continually perpetuates itself because of the unity of form between memory and mental permeation.

IV.10 The desire for life is eternal, therefore, mental permeation has no origin.

IV.11 Cause, consequence, mental coloring, and object support are interdependent, and when they disappear, desire ceases to manifest.

IV.12 The past and the future are always potentially present. Their manifestations depend on individual and universal laws as a whole.

IV.13 Whether individual and universal laws manifest or not depends on the three constituent qualities of nature.

IV.14 An object's reality depends on uniting the changes of the three constituent qualities of nature.

IV.15 The psyche's fragmentary nature creates a divergence between the object and one's grasp of it, even though the object itself remains coherent.

IV.16 For an object to exist, the mind need not perceive it. Otherwise, without perception, would there be any objective reality?

IV.17 The mind perceives objects or not, depending on the attraction they exert and the interest one has in them.

IV.18 The spiritual entity is unchanging and always knows and is master of the ever-changing mind.

IV.19 The mind cannot perceive itself as object.

IV.20 And it is impossible to be conscious of the two simultaneously.

IV.21 If consciousness of one's own consciousness originated from another state of consciousness, there would then be infinite regression of phenomena and confusion of memory.

IV.22 When the mind is not turned outward, it reflects consciousness itself.

IV.23 Colored by the spiritual entity that perceives and by what is perceived, the mind manifests all objects.

IV.24 Although diversified by countless latencies, the mind exists on behalf of the higher entity associated with it.

IV.25 One with discerning perception is freed from all searching for the inner being.

IV.26 The mind is then absorbed in discernment, oriented toward serenity.

IV.27 When discernment lapses, disturbing inner mental experiences rush forth due to past permeations.

IV.28 It is said that to abandon these states is to abandon the causes of suffering.

IV.29 Moreover, with complete disinterest even in the higher understanding born of meditation, regardless of time, place, or circumstances, discernment brings contemplation borne on a cloud of virtuous harmony.

IV.30 Then, on this level, all action based on afflictions has vanished.

IV.31 Then knowledge is more or less infinite, all impurity has been repulsed, and little remains to be known.

IV.32 Then, for the constituent qualities of nature, their end is accomplished and their unfolding ceases.

IV.33 The succession of moments appears in the grasp of past and future changes correlative to the next moment.

IV.34 In liberation, the play of the constituent qualities of nature is no longer a source of meaning or interest to the spiritual entity, or, liberation is the supreme power of pure consciousness founded on itself. End.

CHAPTER I

CONTEMPLATION

sadhānapādaḥ

CONTEMPLATION

Why is method (discussed in Chapter II) introduced after aim (discussed in Chapter I)?

What should we infer from this?

Before beginning, do I believe that pursuing this goal will, in itself, give me the energy I need to reach it?

Chapter I is for those ready to enter the contemplative stage more directly. Contemplation is presented as a progressive means of union with the chosen object, then as a state of transparency difficult to render in words.

This first chapter can be summarized in one question: What is yoga and how do we practice and apply it? The aphorisms answer this question in all its aspects.

I.1 to I.4	What is yoga?
I.5 to I.11	What is the mind?
I.12 to I.29	How can we attain the yoga state?
I.30 to I.31	What difficulties might we encounter?
I.32 to I.39	How can we overcome them?
I.40 to I.51	What does yoga bring us?

samādhipādaḥ
samādhi-pāda

Samdhi: contemplation, union, totality, accomplishment, final achievement. *Pda:* chapter, the foot, the quarter.

I.1

Now is set forth authoritative teaching on yoga.

How do I feel about the sutras, their origins, and their manner of transmission?

What preliminary steps lead me to this study?

Can I openly question the text in a way that does not cast doubt on it?

The first term (*atha*) of the first sutra refers to God, represented by the letter a. In the *Bhagavad Gītā,* the Lord says: I am the *A* of the alphabet (*B. G.*X.33). The meaning of *God* will gradually grow clearer; here it implies a respectful attitude toward yoga.

Atha also refers to the preliminary step a disciple takes to study this text. Auspices are good once this step has been taken; the master reckons the disciple is ready.

Yoga teaching is founded on living experience and continuity in the oral tradition (*anu*). Since yoga is based on direct experience, not written knowledge, it is irrefutable (*śās*).

Here the word *yoga* cuts across the welter of different meanings available; it is both the means of attaining the yoga state and the state itself.

One of the classical commentators, *Vyāsa,* lists five personality types:

- people prey to frantic agitation
- forgetful, amorphous people incapable of controlling their sensuality
- halfway types, alternatively capable of thoughtful reflection or of plunging once more into doubt and inertia
- people endowed with a good capacity of concentration and showing deep interest for all authentic endeavors
- people whose mind is at peace and totally under the control of the being

Yoga allows one to progress, especially from the halfway state to the superior levels.

atha yogānuśānam
atha yoga-ānuśānam

Atha: here and now. *Yoga:* of yoga. *Anuśānam:* outline, teaching, doctrine.

Yoga is the ability to direct and focus mental activity.

Does my practice really transform how I think?

If so, how and in which spheres?

How much do I apply yoga to my daily life?

Through yoga, can I become more aware of what I am and what I am doing?

Yoga consists of keeping the mind quiet and wakeful so that one is totally present to what one is doing. Thoughts no longer rush forth of themselves in all directions, but are fully controlled and directed.

The word mind here is taken in a very large sense. It is the psyche, intelligence, thought, sentiment, and emotion, whether in the conscious or the unconscious.

In the yoga state, mental activities which were previously a source of disturbance are submerged by a stronger, more harmonious, more correct state of mind which is directed at will.

This major aphorism defines yoga and specifies its limits. It concerns the mind, its activities and fluctuations, which often cause human suffering. It aims to alleviate suffering through purifying and harmonizing the mind.

The other aphorisms will not be properly understood unless they are approached in relation to this one.

yogaścittavṛttinirodhaḥ
yogaḥ citta-vṛtti-nirodhaḥ

Yoga: yoga. *Citta:* of the psyche, mind, intelligence, thought, sentiments, emotions. *Vṛtti:* of fluctuations, movements, activities, and modes of functioning (of the mind). *Nirodhaḥ:* stopping, controlling.

With the attainment of focused mind, the inner being establishes itself in all its reality.

How can we know that we are perceiving reality through the inner being? What makes others recognize this in someone?

What is the role of self-knowing in the yoga state?

With serenity, can I see myself as I really am?

Is a total absence of subjectivity possible?

What qualities must I develop for my true nature to unfold?

This aphorism further defines yoga by describing the yoga state. The next aphorism reminds us of our ordinary state of mental fluctuation. Yoga affirms that it is possible to live at a higher level of consciousness where our grasp on reality is pure, total, and absolute, without mental projections.*

Our thoughts and words represent the truth; our inner dimension relates directly to the outer world without mind-distorting perceptions.

We translate *draṣṭar* as inner being. The word *draṣṭar* comes from the root *dṛṣ*—see, perceive, observe, or contemplate. Use of this root reveals two interdependent aspects of ourselves:

- an inner dimension that is absolute (*draṣṭar*), with fullness of knowledge and beatitude, that perceives and experiences
- a relatively outer level that manifests as the body, the mind, and the psyche (*dṛśyam*).

There can be no perception without the manifestation of the object or the presence of the seeing entity. This higher level of consciousness is man's true nature, freed at that moment from its old conditioning, like a butterfly breaking out of its chrysalis.

tadā draṣṭuḥ svarūpe 'vasthānam
tadā draṣṭuḥ svarūpe-avasthānam

Tadā: then. *Draṣṭuḥ:* of the inner being, of the seeing entity, of the witness (from *dṛś:* see, perceive, contemplate). *Svarūpe:* in its true shape, in its true nature. *Avasthānam:* the establishment, setting in place.

*Here the word projection is used in one of its psychoanalytic senses, in which the subject perceives in the outer world, and particularly in others, traits that are actually the subject's own.

Otherwise, we identify with the activities of the mind.

How much do I project my own characteristics unto others?

How important are the outer aspects of personality, such as social standing, family, and professional responsibilities?

What are the ramifications of always seeking greener grass (for example, geographically, professionally, or in our relationships) instead of living fully where we are?

How can we avoid being overly tempted to imitate others?

In our ordinary, scattered state of mind, vision is subjective and partially distorted and thus causes suffering to some degree.

We play parts like actors on a stage, identifying with the characters we are interpreting. We are tossed about and carried away by events and the whirlpool of our mind.

Self-identification with the difficulties we encounter tends to make us dramatize them and lose track of what is really going on.

How many of us see only the negative side of our experience, always somehow dissatisfied with sex life, profession, family situation, marital status, children, other activities, and even our mental and physical make-up? And how many of us think others are enjoying the advantages we lack (*itaratra*)?

Here our thoughts become strongly linked with imagination and misperception.

vṛttisārūpyamitaratra
vṛtti-sārūpyam-itaratra

Vṛtti: mental (activity). *Sārūpyam:* identification, that which has the same form, that which is like. *Itaratra:* otherwise, elsewhere, without which.

I.5

Mental activities are of five kinds, whether they produce suffering or not.

Does my mind help me draw nearer to the yoga state, or does it carry me away?

How do mental activities (listed in the next aphorism) influence my behavior:

- *Does what I notice distract me or inform me?*
- *Do I prefer daydreaming to active creativity?*
- *Do I use my memory to fantasize or to learn?*

Do I use my mind to draw closer to the divine or to drift away from it?

The yoga just defined as a higher state of mind is described in aphorisms I.5 to I.11. Patañjali lists five mental activities. Other authors or systems find fewer or more; Patañjali's choice is simple and complete.

As yoga aims to reduce human suffering, it helps us to see the mind in its relationship to suffering. The mind is like a river that can flow in either of two directions: that of unhappiness (*pāpam*) which gives rise to suffering, and that of happiness (*kalyanakta*). Any mental activity can cause suffering or not, depending on the individual and on circumstances.

Mental activities provoke suffering when they separate us from the yoga state. They reduce suffering when they draw us nearer to that state. Thus, we should not look upon mental activity as good or bad in itself.

vṛttayaḥ pañcatayya kliṣṭākliṣṭāḥ
vṛttayaḥ pañcatayyaḥ kliṣṭa-akliṣṭāḥ

Vṛttayaḥ: (mental) activities. *Pañcatayyaḥ:* of five kinds. *Kliṣṭa:* producing suffering, painful, distressing. *Akliṣṭāḥ:* not producing suffering, not painful, not distressing.

The five mental activities are: understanding, error, imagination, deep sleep, and memory.

In each of us, does one of these mental activities predominate?

Do temperament, profession, family, geography, or other people influence this predilection?

Am I more inclined toward:

- *clearsightedness and understanding, or making mistakes?*
- *inventiveness and creativity, or living in a dream-world, half asleep?*
- *learning useful things by heart, or burdening myself with conventional ideas?*

Is predominance of one of these mental activities beneficial?

To what extent can I choose the mental activity most suitable for a given situation and maintain that mindset?

Here the five mental activities are described:

- Understanding, or correct mental grasp, is a mode of apprehension, of measuring reality (*mā:* to measure).
- Error appears to be correct grasp, but is actually a misunderstanding that originates either from the information itself or from its bad transmission, reception, or interpretation.
- Imagination is the faculty of creating things that do not correspond with reality, but with no pejorative connotation.
- Deep sleep is dreamless sleep. It differs from the dreamlike state (*svapna*) introduced in aphorism I.38.
- Memory is the faculty of recording elements that issue from the other four activities. In spite of the similarity (IV.9) in the way memory and latent impressions (I.17) work, memory is first and foremost mental.

Personality stems from the five activities—from their hierarchical structure, and from the way they have been used. It is influenced by atavism, heredity, and all the past inscribed in the psyche and conditioned behaviors.

In practicing yoga, we seek to:

- develop a correct mental grasp that influences our evolution in a positive way
- reduce mistakes that cause suffering, even though they may galvanize us to activity, fresh questioning, or improved attitude

- use the imagination creatively, as it is the basis of all creation, artistic or otherwise
- respect the restful sleep that is indispensable for regenerating our being
- use the knowledge of what issues from the other four mental activities in a positive way

The mind must be in union with the inner being (*draṣṭar*), with proper consciousness and life of its own. Without this, the mind is an inanimate instrument, because it belongs to the second entity in our being (*dṛśyam*). Like the body, it is made of matter—its life comes to it from another plane.

The aphorisms that follow discuss the five mental states.

pramāṇaviparyayavikalpanidrāsmṛtayaḥ
pramāña-viparyaya-vikalpa-nidrā-smṛtayaḥ

Pramāṇa: correct mental grasp, understanding, real knowledge. *Viparyaya:* error. *Vikalpa:* imagination, ideation. *Nidrā:* deep (dreamless) sleep. *Smṛtayaḥ:* memory.

Understanding arises from sensory perception, inference, and faithful testimony.

In seeking understanding, do I tend more toward:

- *placing my confidence in someone else's experience?*
- *analyzing my experience?*
- *firmly believing in my own experience?*

Does personal evolution always proceed from the teacher's (or another's) testimony to an intellectual understanding and then to direct experience?

Might this order vary according to temperament, age, experience, sociological or cultural surroundings, or the era?

What are the effects in daily life of an attitude (advised by yoga) that favors direct experience in one's relationships with others and with oneself?

Correct mental grasp or understanding (*pramāṇa*) orginates from three activities:

- Sensory perception, dependent on the five senses, is a means of direct self knowledge. Perception is exterior, material, and objective (*laulika*) when it applies to perception outside the body. It is interior and immaterial (*alaulika*) when it is concerned with such sensations as body aches or sentiments. The word *pratyākṣa* implies that the subject, interested in an object, moves toward it and perceives it as long as there are no obstacles.
- Mental grasp, or inference, is indirect knowledge. We use it when we cannot perceive the object with our senses. It includes modes of reflection and analysis—induction, deduction, and so on. The subject is the only one to interpret the message received through mental grasp.
- Testimony is also indirect—that passed via a third person. Although it applies to any testimony, the word *āgamā* primarily designates the sacred texts, both written and orally translated. It concerns the testimony of someone who is an authority in the matter.

Yoga emphasizes sensory perception, unlike other systems of thought, which lean more on sacred texts or induction and analysis.

It is difficult to conceive of one of these three modes of mental grasp, or understanding, apart from the other two. Is it possible, for example, to recognize an object without instantly comparing it with other objects? Doesn't this depend on training and education, and therefore on testimony? Furthermore, is this distinction between the three origins of understanding a little artificial? Not really. Though each of these three modes of apprehending reality is specific, with its own shade of difference, the three are interdependent.

pratyakṣānumānāgamāḥ pramāṇāni
pratyakṣā-numāna-āgamāḥ pramāṇāni

Pratyakṣa: sensory perception. *Anumāna:* inference, induction, deduction. *Āgamāḥ:* testimony worthy of faith, revelation. *Pramāṇāni:* correct mental grasp.

Error is incorrect knowledge based on misinterpretation of reality.

Isn't error a way of hiding from my illusions about myself?

Is this a source of suffering? How can I reduce it?

Can I use error to help prevent future suffering?

Am I ready to learn the error of my ways and take a leap forward?

Is a happy life one in which I:

- *don't make mistakes?*
- *make few grave errors?*
- *am able to look on the bright side of each event?*

When I catch myself making a mistake, how can I use it to enhance my growth?

Misperception is often due to drawing a hasty conclusion while in the grip of emotions. The fable of the snake and the stick is relevant here: To avoid what he took for a snake, but which was really only a stick, a man threw himself into a ditch where he was bitten by a scorpion.

Even though error is false knowledge, it anchors firmly in the mind. It derives from the obstacles set out in the seventh verse of the authoritative text of the *Sāṃkhya,* the *Sāṃkhya-kārikā:* an object too far or too near, infirmity of the senses, inattention, an object too small, hidden, overshadowed by, or mingled with other similar objects.

A distorted view of ourselves and of others is common. It is rooted in automatisms and prejudices, and can only be recognized by hindsight. How can we simultaneously make a mistake and excuse ourselves for it?

Not always negative, error can lead us to question ourselves once more and to progress. Truth is often a succession of corrected mistakes.

Yoga aims at discovering and reducing the causes of misperception in order to diminish suffering.

viparyayo mithyājñānamatadrūpapratiṣṭham
viparyayaḥ mithyā-jñānam-atad-rūpa-pratiṣṭham

Viparyayaḥ: error, mistake. *Mithyā:* incorrect, false. *Jñānam:* knowledge, learning. *A-tad-rūpa:* on a form different from what it really is. *Pratiṣṭham:* based, established.

Imagination is knowledge based on words that have no real, corresponding object.

Do I often live in the imaginary?

What part does imagination play in my daily life?

Does my profession leave room for imagination?

Do I use imagination for creativity or to flee from reality?

Can it be said that imagination is negative when it cuts us off from reality, and that it is positive when it helps create a new reality?

How can we learn to better use imagination?

Imagination uses thought to create nonexistent realities. An architect walking over the land creates a house in his or her mind. A composer writing pages of musical notes hears a symphony in the heart. Although it cannot be seen in the surroundings, imagination lets us glimpse reality in ourselves.

Using imagination, we can represent abstract concepts as well as create new things by associating elements of nature.

Where oral tradition predominates, imagination expresses whole worlds through verbal transmission of ideas. In a society where the visual and the aural predominate, images and sounds flower in the imagination.

Imagination is founded on immediate perceptions, on the contents of memory, and on their interaction. It is at the origin of all artistic creation, such as in eloquent speeches and fine phrases that draw whole crowds in their wake. Imagination helps create life, thus is indispensable to it. But it also can separate us from life.

śabdajñānnupātī vastuśūnyo vikalpaḥ
śabda-jñāna-anupātī vastu-śūnyaḥ vikalpaḥ

Śabda: word, verb, speech, sound. *Jñāna:* knowledge, learning. *Anupātī:* formed of, following from. *Vastu:* of an object, of reality, of matter, of substance. *Śūnyaḥ:* empty, unoccupied, deserted. *Vikalpaḥ:* imagination, ideation.

Deep sleep is a state of unconscious mental activity in which the four other mental activities are eclipsed.

How important is sleep in my daily life?

How can I judge its quality?

Can I be conscious of:

- *the moment when I fall asleep?*
- *the quality of my sleep while I am sleeping?*
- *the nearness of the moment of waking?*

How do sleep, daily activities, and my ability to focus influence each other?

What encourages sound sleep: meals, physical activity, intellectual work, surroundings, human relations, or all of these?

Different from dreaming, deep sleep is qualified by mental passivity and characterized by the absence of other mental activities: understanding, error, imagination, and memory. We may judge its quality by how it influences these activities.

Deep sleep is a time lapse we are conscious of only in retrospect. It is indispensable for recharging our batteries—our vital energy. Indeed, great masters affirm that we return temporarily to God during deep sleep. They explain that after a good night's sleep, we feel refreshed not from physiological rest, but from the fresh energy that flows to us from God. This energy nourishes the spiritual, psychological, and physical levels of the human being.

In this way, deep sleep is like the state of meditation (cf. notably I.38), but with at least one notable difference: in sleep we are not conscious of phenomena, while during meditation we are fully conscious of them.

abhāvapratyayālambanā tamovṛttirnidrā
abhāva-pratyaya-ālambanā tamaḥ-vṛttiḥ-nidrā

Abhāva: absence. *Pratyaya:* experience, the contents of the mind. *Ālambanā:* support, stay. *Tamaḥ:* inertia, incomprehension, torpor, unconsciousness. *Vṛttiḥ:* fluctuation, the way (the mind) functions. *Nidrā:* deep sleep.

I.11

Memory retains living experience.

How does memory affect my daily life and my relationships with others?

Do I need reminder notes to express myself or to go shopping?

Is memory more of an instrument or an obstacle for my personality or my evolution (in yoga, for example)?

Am I better at remembering perceived realities, errors and faults, or fantasies and dreams?

How does the capacity, adaptability, and reliablility of memory change during the course of life?

How does society and the age I live in condition my memory?

What causes loss of memory?

How can I improve my memory?

Do I remember and memorize most easily by phrases, images, or both?

Memory recaptures living experience or prevents it from escaping, often assisted by the other four mental activities

True memory should be exact and its contents consistent with lived experience. It is impossible, however, to differentiate the sources of a memory—perception, analysis during integration, and imagination.

While memory is indispensable to progress (I.20), it can also be an obstacle, or screen, to perception, because it is linked to prejudice, cultural conditioning, and our own desires.

According to the tenets of Āyurvedic medicine, memory's wellspring is in the heart. The more one loves, the better one remembers. Thus, we say "learn by heart."

anubhūtaviṣayāsapramoṣaḥ smṛti'ḥ
anubhūta-viṣaya-asaṃpramṣoaḥ smṛtiḥ

Anubhūta: lived, perceived experience. *Viṣaya:* of the object, of the field of action, of the object of sensory experience. *Asaṃpramṣoaḥ:* the fact of remembering, retention without loss. *Smṛtiḥ:* memory.

Control over the mind's fluctuations comes from persevering practice and nonattachment.

Am I capable of persevering in a real search for a superior level of attention?

And for that, am I ready to detach myself from all the rest?

Also, can I avoid being overcommitted to my endeavor?

Am I better suited to persevering practice or to developing nonattachment?

Can an excess of one weaken the other?

To what extent does persevering practice help or hinder my daily life?

To what extent can nonattachment present a help or a hindrance in daily life?

How can we balance not doing enough, doing things well, and overdoing things?

Aphorism I.2 has already proposed the yoga state as a way to control the five mental activities, defined in aphorisms I.7 through 1.11.

The etymology of the Sanskrit word *abhyāsa* designates persevering practice, which implies intensity, brave encounter, and always persevering with the same impulse in the chosen direction. This practice is defined in the next two aphorisms.

In the context of this chapter, persevering practice primarily designates an inner state of great stability. Posture practice (holding and repeating postures), breathing, and any exercise of physical concentration are to be done to support this state.

For the believer, persevering practice is a continual effort to focus attention and direct it toward the spiritual dimension of being and the creator. From this attitude, nonattachment follows.

Nonattachment (*vairāgya*) signifies the stability and serenity that arise when we withdraw from passion. The less we identify with our passions, the greater is our innter peace, in spite of difficulties. Nonattachment implies freedom with regard to affects, emotions, and sentiments.

Persevering practice is a way of proceeding, and nonattachment is what comes of it. They are interdependent, forming an indissociable pair, linked through their complementarity.

On the one hand, persevering practice or one's commitment to a path, implies detaching oneself from other paths. On the other hand, attachment to the chosen path should also be avoided. One should detach oneself from the practice as something in itself, though all the while pursuing it.

The use of the dual ablative (*abhyām:* origin) stresses the indissoluability of a couple, implying a tight link between perseverance and nonattachment. The two means are as interdependent as needle and thread to sew with, or ink and pen for writing. If one of the pair is missing, there is nothing to be done.

For one persevering with intense practice in spite of obstacles, nonattachment brings peace of mind and calm, allowing one to relax, perfectly at ease and without tensions.

abhyāsavairāgyābhyāṃ tannirodhaḥ
abhyāsa-vairāgyābhyāṃ tad-nirodhaḥ

Abhyāsa: by way of persevering practice. *Vairāgyābhyām:* by way of nonattachment, noninvolvement. *Tad:* of these (fluctuations). *Nirodhaḥ:* stopping, control.

Persevering practice is the effort to attain and maintain the state of mental peace.

Am I ready to try to remain stable and serene in the face of adversity and countercurrents?

Can I work toward and maintain a peaceful mind at all times in the course of my daily life, or is this possible only through an effort of will?

How does inner stability benefit my actions?

As the mind becomes more stable, does action become more instantaneous, precise, and even spontaneous?

How can we keep our control over fluctuation from hampering spontaneity?

Persevering practice allows us to turn a calm and serene mind at will in the chosen direction. Great vigilance is necessary if we are to avoid all deviations. It is this great vigilance that we call effort or zeal.

With this effort, we do not frustrate, repress, or manipulate (*manu militari*) our negative impulses, rather we engage in a progressive and intelligent apprenticeship that keeps us on our toes, whatever the adverse currents or disastrous tendencies may be.

It implies renewed questioning of the many elements of our environment, such as the food we eat, our relationships, our activities, or even ourselves.

It means steering a straight course with neither too little nor too much energy, in spite of the continually eddying currents of our personal leanings and outside circumstances.

It goes without saying that the beginner in navigation should follow the advice of the experienced helmsman.

tatra sthitau yatno'bhyāsaḥ
tatra sthitau yatnaḥ-abhyāsaḥ

Tatra: there, in that case. *Sthitau:* in stability, the establishment. *Yatnaḥ:* tenacious effort. *Abhyāsaḥ:* persevering practice.

I.14

Such a practice is firmly established only if one engages in it seriously and respectfully over a long and uninterrupted period.

Do I have the patience to wait for a long-term results?

How can I prevent interruptions from interfering with my course?

Is yoga a leisure pursuit, or something I take up heart and soul?

Do I organize my practice according to my life, or my life according to my practice?

Am I dealing with innate qualities or with means to acquire and develop them?

Are some qualities more important than others, according to different temperaments? Is it enough just to have these qualities?

Does this aphorism teach a personal way to proceed?

For teachers, does it teach how to choose students and set objectives for them?

The fundamental qualities of persevering practice allow attainment of steadiness and a greater stability of mind. Persevering practice deeply tranforms character and behavior. One does not change just for a few days; long duration and continuity are necesary. All prolonged interruption is an obstacle that diminishes motivation and the qualities acquired. Continuity reflects the respect already introduced by the first letter of the text (I.1) the *a* of *atha.* One should engage in yoga with all one's being (*satkāra*) and offer oneself completely (*ādara*).

The battle is not yet won! But, at least one's way of proceeding is built on solid foundations that will weather the storms raised by personal difficulties, sickness, and old age.

sa tu dīrghakālanairantaryasatkārādarāsevito dṛḍhabhūmiḥ
saḥ tu dīrgha-kāla-nairantarya-satkāra-dara-āsevitaḥ dṛḍha-bhūmiḥ

Saḥ: this, the latter (persevering practice). *Tu:* but, however. *Dīrgha:* long. *Kāla:* for a certain time, duration. *Nairantarya:* without interruption, with continuity. *Satkāra:* with seriousness, rectitude, reverence. *Ādara:* with respect, zeal, care. *Āsevitaḥ:* nourished by, frequented by. *Dṛḍha:* firm. *Bhūmiḥ:* foundation, ground.

Nonattachment is the mastery of desire for perceived external objects, as well as for internal spiritual objects, heard or revealed.

Do I tend to be attached to, or detached from, sensual, affective, or sexual experiences? What conclusions can I draw from this?

Am I attracted, or even attached, to the invisible universe of inner, spiritual, and mystical endeavors? How can this help me?

Is it better to develop nonattachment by acknowledging desires or by letting them pass in silence?

Can experiencing the good things in life help us to detach from them—without running away from them?

Does replacing excessive attachment to visible things with a provisional attachment to the subtle universe further my development of nonattachment?

In a moment of action, what freedom can such nonparticipation give?

Nonattachment is explained in connection with two distinct spheres: seen objects and heard objects. These terms have very wide meanings. Traditionally, the term *seen* (*dṛṣṭa*) designates the entire sphere of the visible world, that is, what the sense organs perceive. This is the profane world, the outer one. The word *heard* (*anuśravika*) represents that which is transmitted by oral tradition or through revealed knowledge. This is the inner world, the sacred one, the heavenly universe.

Nonattachment is, therefore, the conscious realization that all desires provoked by outer and inner objects and realities are under control of the will. It is then that moderation shows itself.

Exterior objects and realities comprise material and intellectual goods as a whole, for example, food, possessions, and intellectual knowledge. The inner world is the one of spiritual endeavor. So, one must be above all desire, including desire concerning mystical sensations or states, or any parapsychological phenomenon.

Someone prone to strong attachment, for example, dependent on tobacco or alcohol, frequently becomes attached to religious commitments or a yoga practice. The result is an excess of one or the other, sometimes to the detriment of health and a balanced personality. Even though the new attachments are less destructive than the first and progress is certain, the difficulty is not yet resolved, simply displaced.

That nonattachment follows persevering practice (I.12) points out the means of discovering it. The result of exerting effort or will can be repression or frustration rather than nonattachment. Through nonattachment we consciously realize that attachment to any object can create short or long-term negative effects of dependency that weaken physical and mental stability and strength. Nonattachment does not mean detaching oneself from things, but discovering that things drop away of themselves.

dṛṣṭānuśravikaviṣayavitṛṣṇasya vaśīkrasaṃjñāvairāgyam
dṛṣṭa-ānuśravika-viṣaya-vitṛṣṇasya vaśīkra-saṃjñā-vairāgyam

Dṛṣṭa: seen, the visible universe, perceptible, *Ānuśravika:* heard, revealed inner universe, tradition. *Viṣaya:* for objects. *Vitṛṣṇasya:* of the absence of desire. *Vaśīkāra:* of mastery, submission to the will. *Saṃjñā:* consciousness, the fact of becoming perfectly conscious. *Vairāgyam:* nonattachment.

At its highest level, nonattachment means having no desire for any of the constituent qualities of nature, because one has become conscious of the spiritual principle.

Am I always aware of an inner presence that shapes my thoughts, my words, and my actions, and sustains the state of nonattachment?

How do I avoid confusing nonattachment with indifference?

How do I stay detached, yet motivated?

How do I reconcile the distinctive character of the constituent qualities of nature with complete detachment from them?

Does such higher nonattachment help or hinder action?

Is the way we feel about death related to how attached we are to the physical body and life?

The highest level of nonattachment emerges from a spiritual dimension designated by the word *puruṣa*. In this particular text *puruṣa* is a principle that represents:

- permanent as opposed to temporary
- spirit as opposed to matter
- absolute as opposed to relative
- essence as opposed to existence

Puruṣa is practically synonymous with the word *draṣṭar*, translated as inner being in aphorism I.3. It is eternal, individual, and has no attributes, unlike matter and its constituent qualities.

The Vedic tradition introduces the concept of constituent qualities of nature (*guṇas*), defined and explained in the *Sāṃkya-Kārikā* and illustrated by a series of concrete examples in the *Bhagavad Gītā* (sacred text serving as the popular basis for Hinduism). Life manifests as a mixture of the three fundamental qualities. Each object, each temperament, each mood of an instant, is a mixture of these three qualities or attributes. No object can appear, for example, without mixing of the qualities of nature that manifest as color, density, weight, and volume.

Patañjali and Kapila respectively in the *Yoga-sutrā* and the *Sāṃkhya-Kārikā* use different words to designate these three fundamental qualities:

Yoga:		Sāmkhya:	
śīla	*Qualities*	*Guṇa*	*Qualities*
prakāśa	understanding	*sattva*	clarity
kriyā	movement	*rajas*	activity
sthiti	inertia	*tamas*	obscurity

Supreme nonattachment is not the result of a decision, but emerges from a mystical state. The qualities of the outer world do not disappear, but lose their power of attraction. This higher degree of nonattachment widens the domain of seen and heard objects (I.15) to embrace the constituent qualities of nature as a whole.

At this level of nonattachment, merely suppressing desire is not enough. There comes to be an absence of thirst for the qualities or the psychological states of inertia and activity, or even for the state of clarity.

Such nonattachment exists in one to whom a higher presence has been revealed. This higher inner presence makes worldly attractions appear quite relative. It is the revelation of the spiritual principle that leads to the absence of thirst, rather than the absence of thirst leading to this revelation. This higher nonattachment is a marked sign of spiritual evolution, the state of the great mystics and poets who sing God's praises.

tatparaṃ puruṣakhytergunavaitṛṣṇyam
tat-paraṃ purua-khyāteḥ-guṇa-vaitṛṣṇyam

Tat: this, the former (nonattachment). *Param:* extreme, supreme, at (to) its highest degree. *Puruṣa:* of the spiritual principle (inherent in every one). *Khyāteḥ:* (because of) the awareness (becoming aware). *Guṇa:* for the constituent qualities of nature, the attribute, the property (*sattva:* understanding; clarity; rajas: movement, activity; tamas: inertia, incomprehension, obscurity). *Vaitṛṣṇyam:* absence of desire.

Perfect contemplation with full consciousness of the object passes, becoming reflective contemplation, then intuitive, then beatific, and lastly, full consciousness of self in the experience.

Am I ready to immerse myself in an object—for example, an idea of work or a human relationship—to feel its reality in the depths of myself as though I, personally, no longer exist?

Am I able to reach this high level of relationship with any object? If not, is it just attachment?

Am I better able to realize this state:

- *with eyes closed, using a theme of reflection?*
- *with eyes wide open in an activity?*
- *in relationships with others?*

Can we conceive of beatitude without being fully conscious of existence?

According to Patañjali, there are two categories of sentiment: that which permits deep understanding and beatitude; and that which chains us to suffering (II.6). How can we distinguish between them?

Persevering practice and nonattachment prepare the mind to pass from mental dispersion toward contemplation on an object. This contemplation passes through four chronological stages.

Contemplation is not a state of emptiness or nothingness—far to the contrary. In contemplation one perceives deep reality—the essence of the object—which serves as a starting point for meditation.

At this level of perfect orientation, the mind first grasps the object through a process of reflection and analysis that uses memory, words, and images free of the distorting interference of personality. This is the first approach to an object. It permits general understanding (*vitarka*).

This is followed by a more intuitive grasp of a surprising nature that seems to come from a deeper space (*vicāra*). Then, this knowledge and experience flood one with joy, or beatitude (*ānanda*), and one becomes quite conscious of being fully alive (*asmitā*). This individual consciousness is no longer egocentric nor individualistic—it transcends individuality.

Patañjali uses the same word to describe individual consciousness (*asmitā*), whether it brings joy or suffering (II.3 and II.6) shaped by egoism. There can be only one individual state of consciousness at a time. Its source is the spiritual entity, or the inner being (*draṣṭar*), the perception of which the mind veils or not. If transparent, individual consciousness is correct; if clouded, it is egocentric.

In these successive states of union with an object, consciousness does not change. The mind of the person becomes more and more transparent, until consciousness reflects the object of contemplation with purity.

vitarkavicārānandāsmitārūpnugamātsaṃprajñātaḥ
vitarka-vicāra-ānandā-asmitā-rūpa-anugamāt-saṃprajñātaḥ

Vitarka: of reasoning. *Vicāra:* concerning the subtle, intuitive grasp, reflection. nanda: of beatitude, felicity, joy. *Asmitā:* of consciousness of "I," sentiment of existing. *Rūpa:* form. *Anugamāt:* following, passing by. *Saṃprajñātaḥ:* contemplation with consciousness of an object.

Regular immersion in contemplation without mental fluctuation brings contemplation in which only mental permeation subsists.

What type of personality is most apt to experience this state?

What qualities can prepare me for this state?

What is the relationship between this kind of contemplation and supreme detachment (I.16)?

This kind of contemplation is instantaneous and manifests great peace, clarity, and compassion that takes hold of you.

It is beyond and superior to the preceding state of contemplation with an object. It occurs unexpectedly after being immersed over the years in contemplation with an object, and after persevering practice to stop the wandering mind. The believer attributes it to divine grace.

The expression mental permeation (*saṁskāra**) introduces an important concept in yoga. It can mean make perfect, which refers to conscious and unconscious conditioning. Yoga differentiates between two kinds of mental permeation: that which results from negative impulses (II.15), and that which is positive and stems from the practice of yoga (I.50 and III.10). Yoga is the source of this second kind of contemplation, which is a transitory state. *Kaivalya* (Chapter IV) designates the permanent state.

virāmapratyayābhyāsapūrvaḥ saṃskāraśeṣo nyaḥ
virāma-pratyaya-abhyāsa-pūrvaḥ saṃskāra-śeṣaḥ-anyaḥ

Virāma: concerning the cessation, renouncing. *Pratyaya:* of mental experience. *Abhyāsa:* persevering practice. *Pūrvaḥ:* preceded by. *Saṃskāra:* mental residue from past acts, mental permeation. *Śeṣaḥ:* the remainder. *Anyaḥ:* the other (kind of contemplation).

**Saṁskāra* 1) perfecting, refining, polishing; 2) refinement, perfection, grammatical purity (as of words); 3) education, cultivation, training (as of the mind); 4) making ready, preparation; 5) cookery, dressing (of food); 6) embellishment, decoration ornament; 7) consecration, sanctification, hallowing; 8) impression, form, mold, operation, influence; 9) idea, notion, conception; 10) any capacity, or faculty; 11) effect of work, merit of action; 12) the self-reproductive quality; 13) The faculty of recollection, impression on the memory; 14) a purification rite, a sacred rite or ceremony; 15) purification, purity; 16) a rite or ceremony in general; 17) investiture with the sacred thread; 18) obsequious ceremony; 19) a polishing stone (from Dict. V.S. APTE).

I.19

This state is innate for two kinds of predestined beings: "those without a body" and "those who are reabsorbed into original matter."

Certain beings, recognized while still quite young, possess great mental clarity and compassion, or elevated spiritual values. What are the advantages and the inconveniences of such privileged birth?

What should one so blessed do with these gifts?

How should we treat those who possess them?

How can one avoid wasting these gifts?

Two kinds of human being may attain this instantaneous contemplation without an object: "those without a body" and "those who are reabsorbed into original matter."

In Hinduism, these two expressions refer to people who attained spiritual freedom in another incarnation and who return to earth to help others. Their interests transcend the body and material goods. The second kind are at a superior level.

This aphorism states that certain people are born with exceptional gifts, however, this does not mean that these gifts are necessarily irrevocable. Aphorisms IV.1 to IV.7 list, in order of value, the origins of powers, and the least considered is birth. The son and heir who receives a fortune without work or obstacles is not always strong enough to use it to advantage. He is easy prey. One may say the same of spiritual values.

For Westerners living in a society marked by Judeo-Christian culture these two categories of beings correspond to exceptional personalities who are born full of wisdom, high intelligence, and compassion.

bhavapratyayo videhaprakṛtilayānām
bhava pratyayaḥ videha-prakṛtilayānām

Bhava: concerning being, of existing. *Pratyayaḥ:* mental experience. *Videha:* without a body, disincarnate. *Prakṛtilayānām:* those subsisting in constituent elements, reabsorbed in original matter.

For the others, faith engenders energy that reinforces the memory, allowing concentration on wisdom.

Am I sufficiently self-confident? How can I reinforce my confidence?

If our parents did not encourage us to become aware of our own value, how can we develop such confidence as adults?

Can real faith exist without energy? And vice versa?

What is the range of values between success that creates positive conditioning, and failure, whose lesson should be retained?

Should a yoga teacher choose a student according to suppleness, intelligence, or confidence?

How does one bolster a child's or a student's confidence?

What is the connection between the idea of confidence and aphorism I.1?

Those not lucky enough to be born in the yoga state can reach it through the qualities listed in this aphorism, which follow a definite order that sets up a cause-and-effect relationship between them.

The word *śraddhā* means "faith in God" and also "self-confidence"—in anybody else or simply in life. The loving confidence that parents create encourages a child to become confident, courageous, and full of energy to act. Where there is no energy, even the names of friends escape us, whereas when full of vitality, memory seems infallible. It allows us to steer a steady course and to avoid repeating the same mistakes. Then concentration and an unswerving direction lead to wisdom.

śraddhāvīryasmṛtisamādhiprajñāpūrvaka itareṣām
śraddhā-vīrya-smṛti-samādhi-prajñā-pūrvakaḥ itareṣām

Śraddhā: faith, conviction. *Virya:* courage, energy, strong will. *Smṛti:* memory, study. *Samādhi:* contemplation, perfect concentration. *Prajñā:* highest knowledge, wisdom. *Pūrvakaḥ:* preceded by, anterior. *Itareṣām:* for others.

I.21

For those impelled by intense ardor, the goal is near.

Am I sufficiently ardent and intense in my undertaking?

How can I keep my enthusiasm from burning out?

How can I reconcile intense ardor with the nonattachment necessary for judicious action?

How can one strengthen a child's ardor or a student's demand?

Is it better to choose students based on their ardor, or the degree of intensity of their demand?

Is it giving more or giving less that strengthens demand?

Yoga is a discipline of individual evolution, and it requires a lot from those who engage in it. It is important to maintain strong motivation. Whatever brings us to yoga, we must sustain it with this intense ardor so that we can overcome the obstacles that will not fail to arise (I.30).

For some, yoga is a necessity, or a calling. From the outset there is urgency—everything else can wait. Their lives revolve around yoga, not the other way around. It is then quite clear that the goal is more rapidly accessible.

Frequently, an Indian master puts his students motives to the test by placing obstacles in their way. He then waits for a demand, and often, for the student to repeat it before responding. In fact, he awakens the ability of his students to take themselves in hand. By doing this he strengthens the student's quest.

tīvrasaṁvegānāmāsannaḥ
tīvra-saṁvegānām-āsannaḥ

Tīvra: intense, ardent. *Saṁvegānām:* impulsion, vehemence. *Āsannaḥ:* near, obtained.

There still remains a difference based on distinct temperaments: gentle, moderate, and lively.

Am I inclined to be tender, gentle, and slow; lively, rapid, and aggressive; or perhaps in between, either alternating between opposing tendencies, or balancing aspects of both?

Can my reactions tell me about my tendencies?

How is this knowledge useful, both personally and in choosing a career, profession, or collaborators?

How can one take this difference into account when teaching several people at the same time?

Is it possible or worthwhile to try to change my temperament or influence that of others?

Motivation and action vary according to temperament. Gentle people are slow to start, level-headed, and thoughtful. They are like the tortoise in the fable. Lively people are impetuous and rapid. They hurtle into action, sometimes with great vivacity, like the hare. Moderate types have an intermediate temperament, at times gentle, at times vivacious.

We can fulfill our goals by recognizing our own temperament and using it to guide our choice of profession, relationships, and leisure pursuits. The ideal is great intensity with level-headedness. We find a broad range of temperaments in the surrounding circle, in which different tendencies create richness in the group. Everybody has a chance perhaps, but it is different for each of us. That is why it is necessary to know and respect everyone's temperament and rhythm—to favor everyone's evolution and allow them to proceed at a rhythm suitable for them. Āyurvedic medicine proposes a precise set of types, described on the following pages.

mṛdumadhyādhimātratvāttato 'pi viśeṣaḥ
mṛdu-madhya-adhimātratvāt-tataḥ-api viśeṣaḥ

Mṛdu: gentle, tender, slow. *Madhya:* middling, intermediary, moderate. *Adhimātratvāt:* (because of the temperament) lively, strong, rapid. *Tataḥ:* following, from then on. *Api:* as well, again. *Viśeṣaḥ:* difference, distinction.

The Three Biological Humors*

The word *prakṛti* means "nature" or "natural form" of the constitution of the body. *Prakṛti* is divided into two main types: physical *prakṛti* (*deha prakṛti or arra prakṛti*) and psychic *prakṛti* (*mnasika prakṛti*). Physical *prakṛti* is classified into three types, or three biological humors (*doṣas*): wind (*vāta prakṛti*), fire (*pitta prakṛti*), and water (*kapha prakṛti*). Of course, these are text book cases. We rarely find a perfect *vāta, pitta,* or *kapha prakṛti.* The overwhelming majority of people are a mixture, with one main type predominating.

THE WIND CONSTITUTION

(v•ta prak®ti)

Vāta is dry, rough, light, mobile, swift, cold, coarse, and nonslimy in quality. Each quality has a specific effect on the formation of *prakṛti*:

- The roughness and dryness of *Vāta* produce rough, dry skin and short stature.
- The lightness of *Vāta* produces light, unsteady movement. This type is frail, wavering, eats lightly, is talkative and speaks quickly, and has similar traits in other activities.
- Mobility produces unstable joints, eyebrows, jaw, lips, tongue, head, shoulder, hands, and feet. *Vāta* persons tend to move their eyebrows, lips, hands, and legs while performing other activities. They have visible joints and tendons and an abundant network of veins visible on hands and legs.
- Swiftness produces hasty initiation of action. They are quick to fear and and to form affections, aversions, or disinclinations. They acquire knowledge quickly, but the memory is poor. They cannot retain for long what they have gained.
- Coldness produces intolerance to cold; they are often afflicted with cold and always feel cold in body, hands, and legs. It also produces stiffness in body.
- Coarseness produces coarse hair, beard, moustache, body hair, nails and teeth, and small face, hands, and feet.
- Nonsliminess produces cracking, sound, and movement in the joints.

Vāta people like sweet, sour, and salty tastes more than the others. They crave warm food and drinks and prefer warm climates, body massage, and sweating. They tend to quarrel with others. Often, they

*This condensed extract is based on the article, "A Few Practical Aspects of the Constitution (Prakṛti)" by Vaida H.S. Kasture, published in *Darshanam,* no. 4.

have dreams of running, jumping, and climbing trees and mountains. Usually, they do not believe others and do not remain trustworthy. They cannot control their passions and therefore are not steady in friendship. They are unstable in mind, gait, and sight, and poor or medium in the sexual act and in the quantity and quality of seminal fluid.

Due to all these qualities, usually they are weak with a short life span, have few progeny, and are short of means and wealth. The development of the body is not properly maintained. Body strength is less, the voice is weak, low, and hoarse, and these people are vigilant.

The Fire Constitution
(*pitta prakṛti*)

Pitta is hot, sharp, liquid, fleshy in smell, sour, and pungent. Each of these qualities has a specific effect in the formation of *prakṛti.*

- Hotness produces intolerance to heat, hot face, and fair and delicate organs. They have plenty of moles, freckles, black moles, pimples, and marks on the skin. They age early, with early appearance of wrinkles and gray hair. They also tend to lose their hair. Their beards and mustaches are sharp, sparse, and brown in color. Body hair is scattered and brown.
- Sharpness produces heroism and valor, courage and strong *agni* (power of digestion). They are always hungry, eating frequently and taking abundant food and plenty of drinks. They cannot undertake sustained, hard work.
- Liquidity produces laxity and softness in joints and muscles, profound sweating, and copious amounts of urine and feces.
- Fleshy smell produces bad smell in the axilla, mouth, head, and body. Pungency and sourness produce insufficient semen, inadequacy in the sexual act, and few progeny.

Pitta Prakṛti people like sweet, astringent, and bitter tastes more than others. They crave cold things, cold foods and drinks. They do not like hot drinks and food. Usually they have dreams of gold, sun, blazing fire, lightning, fiery glow in the sky, fights, quarrels, and struggles. *Pitta* men are not very attractive to women. They are radiant, valorous, proud, irritable with angry natures, fond of disputation in assemblies, difficult to subjugate, show unbending affection toward dependents, and have moderate strength, wealth, means, life span, knowledge, and understanding

The Water Constitution
(kapha prakṛti)

Kapha is unctuous, smooth, soft, sweet, solid, dull, rigid, heavy, cold, slimy, and clear in quality. Each quality produces certain symptoms of *prakṛti* as follows.

- Unctuousness and smoothness produce unctuous and smooth organs.
- Softness produces delicate, fair, and pleasant organs.
- Sweetness produces abundant seminal fluid, strength in the sexual act, and more progeny.
- Essence, or sap quality, produces a compact and stable body. Solidity produces good development of body and of all organs.
- Dullness produces dull and slow activity, food intake, and speech.
- Rigidity produces delayed initiation of action, delayed irritability, and delayed effectiveness.
- Heaviness produces heavy, stable movements.
- Coldness produces very little hunger and thirst, lower body temperature, and little sweating.
- Sliminess produces strong joints and ligaments.
- Clarity produces clear eyes, clear face, and unctuousness on the face and in the voice.

Kapha prakṛti people like pungent, bitter, and astringent tastes. They crave dry and hot things. They dislike humid and cold climates. Their memory is long, but their receptive power is low. They become fearful or excited slowly. Their attachment and detachment is slow. They walk slowly, like a swan, with a stable footing. Their eyes are big and attractive, their arms long and the bones well padded. They have large joints. They have dreams of birds, garlands, swans, rivers, lakes, oceans, and romantic events. They are gentle and God-fearing, and prosperous, self-controlled, merciful, and stable in friendship. Kapha men are loved by women, for they are generous, intelligent, greatly enthusiastic, strong, and have plentiful means, progeny, friends, and wealth.

Otherwise, the goal is attained by active devotion to God.

Can active devotion help me attain the yoga state?

If so, what sort of daily, individual, or group ritual can help me?

Can a believer who feels that he or she harbors the divine presence actively practice devotions outside an established religion?

Can the believer of a particular religious faith venerate the God of his or her religion in a yoga practice?

As devotion is not here a priori, but a means amongst others, what is the difference between yoga and religion?

Since the aphorism starts with "otherwise," is belief really indispensable to the practice of yoga?

Can this aphorism encourage a nonbeliever to accept that we can never master everything, and thus take an important evolutionary step forward?

How can a yoga teacher know when to propose this aphorism to a student and when to wait?

For many Hindu yogis, this aphorism is the most important one. It is difficult for them to conceive of yoga, a mystical path, without religious implications. Some people affirm that the *Yoga Sūtras* really begin with this aphorism; that what went before is only introduction.

Aphorisms I.23 to I.29 present active devotion as an alternative to both persevering practice and nonattachment (I.12). It is the second way to attain contemplation. It is neither the first way nor a goal, but is a possibility adapted to the believer. It is active and consists of a set of gestures, words. and rituals to carry out daily, often in front of a representation of the being to whom one is devoted.

The important concept, *Īśvara-praṇidhāna,* is repeated four times in the *Yoga Sūtras* and can be interpreted according to the passage concerned:

- active devotion (I.23)
- an attitude of acceptance in the course of action (II.1)
- positive behavior that stems from a group of daily ritual acts as a whole (II.32 and II.45)

The word *Īśvara* means master, king, husband, highly placed person, and in Hindu tradition, *Īśvara* signifies:

- the one, personal God
- Supreme *Puruṣa,* the dynamic aspect of Brahman, God as Lord of all nature, the cosmic *ātman*
- any god

Īśvara can symbolize God in the personal aspect as each individual perceives it. More concretely, *Īśvara* is one of the gods venerated in temples of *Śiva* (third manifestation of the triple divine form: creation, equilibrium, destruction). According to tradition, yoga takes its origin from *Śiva,* who taught it to his wife *Pārvatī.* It is the same for *Kṛṣṇa* (eighth incarnation (*avatar*) of *Viṣṇu*), who in the *Bhagavad Gītā,* in the guise of the charioteer in the war, teaches yoga not only to *Arjuṇa,* the archer who directs the chariot, but to the army as well. This is also the case for *Viṣṇu,* second divine form, responsible for the equilibrium of the universe.

A reader brought up in the Judeo-Christian culture must guard against taking *Īśvara* as Creator of Heaven and Earth. He represents omniscience, the root of all knowledge, and is the spiritual guide above all others. Thus, a Hindu can include vara in his yoga practice and still pray to the God of his own religion, *Nārāyaṇā,* for example. Yoga has universal value; there is no conflict with religion. Yoga awakens the believer in his or her own religion.

Active devotion is the best way for the believer. All it requires is to abandon oneself and to show devotion with all one's being every day. The Lord does the rest.

īśvarapraṇidhānādvā
īśvara-praṇidhānāt-vā

Īśvara: God, Lord (from *īś:* to be master of, power be able], reign). *Praṇidhānāt:* by particular, active devotion. *Vā:* or else.

God is a supreme being free from all causes of suffering—from actions, their consequences, and all latency.

How can I avoid the failure to recognize myself (the first cause of suffering) in being clear about my motives?

Why does devotion to a supreme being free from all conditioning enable us to attain a state quite beyond the perpetual chain of suffering?

How can I recognize the spiritual being in myself (puruṣa) that is identical with the divine model, though imprisoned by negative conditioning?

Yoga's first concern is to alleviate suffering (*duḥkha*). The expression "causes of suffering" (*kleśa*) means here the mistaken impulses that lead to it (lack of recognition, the ego, attachment, repulsion, fear). These are introduced in Chapter II.When they are at the root of a thought, a word, or an action, they bring painful consequences in the form of other actions that themselves leave traces.

One extraordinary being only is not caught in this chain of suffering: God. God is the spectator of it. Outside the cycle, God is liberation and serves as a point of reference for each individual on the way to liberation. To be set free does not mean one must stop acting, but that one acts in a spontaneous and adapted way (IV.6, 7, 8).

Yoga defines God differently from the *Vedānta* and other schools of Indian thought. God is not the Creator, but a spiritual entity (*puruṣa*) free from all action based on the causes of suffering (*kleśa*). God is the model of that to which human beings aspire, and which certain people achieve. God is like us, but without our imperfections.

kleśakarmavipākāśayairaparamṛṣṭaḥ puruṣaviśeṣa īśvaraḥ
kleśa-karma-vipāka-āśayaiḥ-aparāmṛṣṭaḥ puruṣa-viśeṣaḥ īśvaraḥ

Kleśa: cause of suffering, torment, affliction. *Karma:* action, act. *Vipāka:* result, fruit. *Āśayaiḥ:* permeation, mental deposits in the unconscious, traces. *Aparāmṛṣṭaḥ:* untouched, unaffected. *Puruṣa:* the spiritual principle. *Viśeṣaḥ:* extraordinary, distinct (with a sense of superiority). *Īśvaraḥ:* God.

I.25

God (*Īśvara*) is the unequaled source of all knowledge.

What reflection can this principle inspire in me: There is a supreme force (Īśvara) that knows all, has always known, and is infinitely wise?

How can it change me to believe that a higher entity, "made in God's image," dwells in me and is my true being, though it is veiled by negative conditioning?

Does believing that absolute wisdom exists in everyone change how we perceive ourselves and others?

How does belief that wisdom exists in everyone influence teaching or helpful relationships?

What qualities can make my mind transparent to this wisdom?

To alleviate suffering that stems from painful behavior (II.3) is itself based on a faulty vision of ourselves. Yoga offers us the model of supreme, omniscient being of absolute wisdom, without temporal limits.

God knows and recognizes all. No other knowledge, superior or equal to God's, can exist. God is the fountainhead of all knowledge, whatever its sphere. The word knowledge here does not represent intellectual knowledge, so much as lucidity about oneself, or wisdom.

The "god" of yoga is not beyond all attributes, but is infinite. God is a model for human beings—our essence is an identical spiritual entity. However, we remain inferior nonetheless because we are imprisoned in negative impulses and sentiments and bound by corporeal limits.

For the believer, God is omniscient. Nonbelievers might be inclined to see this as absolute knowledge, a wisdom that transcends human being, but toward which we strive. This comes very close to the famous maxim, attributed to Socrates: "Know thyself and thou shalt know the universe."

tatra niratiśayaṃ sarvajñabījam
tatra niratiśayaṃ sarvajña-bījam

Tatra: in him. *Niratiśayam:* unsurpassed, unequaled. *Sarvajña:* of omniscience. *Bījam:* origin, seed, source.

Unsubjected to time, God is the spiritual guide even for the ancients.

Does my belief that yoga comes from a supreme being modify my attitude to this discipline?

Does this mean:

- *I should accept everything from a yoga teacher?*
- *the teaching never contains the slightest error?*
- *it is wrong to criticize my yoga teacher?*

To what extent does the belief that this teaching proceeds from God affect the teacher's attitude?

Does this reinforce the teacher's confidence in their own judgment or confer greater humility?

Is it possible for a nonbeliever to see a discipline emanating from a higher force in yoga?

Perhaps we should use the word guru with a measure of prudence?

This aphorism develops the theme of a supreme being as the origin of all knowledge and adds the notion of eternity. God's knowledge and wisdom are instantaneous, total, have always been, and always will be.

As the source of all knowledge from the very beginning, God is the source of all teaching handed down by the masters of all disciplines. God is the Master of masters. The Sanskrit term *guru,* translated here as "spiritual guide," can be interpreted as "one who leads from obscurity to light." Tradition refers back from master to master to a supreme being as the origin of yoga, attributing every discovery to God. The respect for this is evident in India, where it is customary to bow down to the *guru* before receiving the teaching. In India, the term *guru* designates any person who transmits wisdom, teaching, or knowledge, or who is the spiritual head of a family.

sa eṣa pūrveṣāmapi guruḥ kālenānavacchedāt
saḥ eṣaḥ pūrveṣām-api guruḥ kālena-anavacchedāt

Saḥ eṣaḥ: it is one who. *Pūrveṣām:* for the ancients, those who came before. *Api:* also, even, again. *Guruḥ:* master, instructor, guide. *Kālena:* through time. *Anavacchedāt:* not being limited or subjected to.

I.27

Its expression is the "sacred syllable."

Can the regular repetition in the mind of a word that designates God help me resolve my difficulties or self-pity, rather than ceaselessly wrestle with them?

If certain people are more visual thinkers, and others are more verbal, to which category do I belong and which category does this method suit?

How important is the word I choose for God?

Why did the ancients avoid saying God's name out loud, preferring to write it? Is this valid today?

The expression "sacred syllable" is precise and unequivocal enough to name God. It is also wide enough to allow each religion to refer to God in its own vocabulary. Patañjali's prudence favors the universal application of his treatise. For a Hindu, sacred syllable means *OṂ,* the name common to all the Hindu branches. It is the most universal of *mantras.* A *mantra* is a mystic, sacred formula, an incantation taken from the *Veda,* meant to be recited aloud, softly, or mentally. It is a word pronounced by God and heard by a Sage.

Continually repeated, it awakens spiritual consciousness. The *mantra* corresponds to the auditory, discursive universe on the speech level. Images correspond to the visual universe at level of the frontal lobe.

The *mantra OṂ* can be chanted aloud. However, its mental repetition is considered deeper—like all *mantras,* it should be recited in inner silence. Thus, in many ancient texts, it is considered too sacred to be written. It does not appear in the *Yoga Sūtras,* and is found only four times in the *Bhagavad Gītā* (VIII.13, IX.17, XVII.23, and XVII.24). According to the *Śiva-Saṃhitā,* there are four yogas, of which the first is *mantra-yoga,* addressed to the least gifted adepts (*Śivas* V. 9-10-11).

tasya vācakaḥ praṇavaḥ
tasya vācakaḥ praṇavaḥ

Tasya: of this one, of God. *Vācakaḥ:* that which signifies, expresses, designates. *Praṇavaḥ:* the sacred syllable.

Repeating the sacred syllable and pondering its meaning lead to its understanding.

Am I sufficiently at peace to use the name of God my religion uses?

If I have received no religious education, how can I develop the attitude of deep respect necessary for the regular practice of mantra?

Since a higher being understands every language, is it all right for me to use words from other languages to refer to God?

Do such words have the same resonance?

How can I avoid excessive attachment or the emotional effervescence that may arise from using a mantra?

The practice of yoga is closely linked to recitation of the *mantra.* This is what Vyāsa affirms in his commentary: "Through the contemplative repetition of *mantras,* yoga will be consolidated, and through yoga the chanting of *mantras* is improved. Through the glory of such chanting and such yoga, the supreme soul is revealed."

A technical term used in Hindu rituals, the word repetition (*japa*) refers to the repetition of a prayer a great many times, for example, 108 times, often with the support of prayer beads.

The technique of chanted repetition is clearly set out in many ancient texts (*Upaniṣads*). We are advised to chant *OṂ* naturally, with humility and respect. For instance, the vowel *O* should last three time units (about three seconds), and the nasalized consonant (*anusvāra*) *Ṃ,* half a unit. A brief silence follows.

The word "signification" (*artha*) represents the qualities, the attributes of the supreme being. Yoga places emphasis on a meaning that represents God's omniscience. To represent omniscience:

- *a* is the first vowel of the Sanskrit alphabet
- *u* is a middle letter
- *m* is the last consonant

A-U-Ṃ thus symbolizes the whole body of knowledge that can be transmitted verbally; the silence that follows manisfests knowledge that is not transmissible verbally. *OṂ* also symbolizes the four *Vedas* that contain all knowledge. It is therefore ultimate knowledge.

Among other interpretations, one of the most frequently quoted concerns God in the aspect of Creator, corresponding to the *Vedānta:*

- *a* is the creation : *Brahmā*
- *u* is conservation: *Viṣṇu*
- *m* is destruction: *Śiva*

A-U-Ṃ corresponds to the manifested universe as a whole; the silence that follows is *Brahman:* neuter, absolute, support for the manifestation. These four represent all that is visible or invisible, the Absolute and the relative. Such symbols cannot correspond to *Īśvara* in yoga, where God is omniscient, but not creator.

The writing of *OṂ* is important in a society that emphasizes visual memory more and more. In the most common alphabet of the Sanskrit language, *devanāgarī, OṂ* is written:

निसेरत सयमबोल फरोम पभ ६५ नि बौोकत्रभ

It is universal, not for any single yoga school. Yoga should respect the beliefs, customs, and religion of each one who practices it.

If any symbol could be said to represent groups in India practicing yoga, it is the masculine (turns clockwise) 卍 or feminine (turns counterclockwise) svastika 卐. The word *svastika* means auspicious. It must be used with prudence in the West since the Nazis used a similar sign.

In the Western alphabet, the correct writing is *OṂ.* To write *AUṂ,* decomposing the *O* to recall its symbolism, is an error, for *AU* is a Sanskrit diphthongized vowel pronounced "a-u."

According to the Indian tradition, the power of a *mantra* is a function of the ascetism of the one who hands it down.

Though less developed and less elaborate than in India, the use of repetitive recitations of a word referring to God also exists in other cultures, for example in Christian mysticism.

tajjapastadarthabhāvanam
tad-japaḥ tad-artha-bhāvanam

Tad: regarding, of, this latter (sacred syllable). *Japaḥ:* repetition. *Tad:* of this latter. *Artha:* signification, essence, aim. *Bhāvanam:* realization.

It is then that one understands the self and gradually clears inner obstacles.

Why believe that active devotion to a superior force can bring me closer to my true nature of joy and wisdom?

Am I able to accept that all issues forth from God's will and that God dwells in me?

How can I attain inner consciousness without flying in the face of external or psychological reality?

How can I distinguish between the disappearance of obstacles and their repression (my refusal to see them)?

Is it possible to discover that obstacles we thought were outside are, in fact, inside us, without feeling reproach?

Does discovering inner obstacles ensure their disappearance?

How can I avoid becoming egocentric about this?

Reciting the sacred syllable leads to certain results linked by cause and effect.

When less enslaved by outside solicitations, consciousness turns inward. It discovers a presence full of peace and self-understanding. We accept seeing ourselves as we are, discovering the profound impulses that feed the field of consciousness and determine behavior. To the extent that they were obstacles, we no longer blow them out of proportion in the mind, which then turns toward a higher force. Such a phenomenon is progressive.

Developing the inner state reduces obstacles. Two opposite effects combine: as we gradually acquire something, little by little, something else disappears.

tataḥ pratyakcetanādhigamo 'pyantarāyābhāvaśca
tataḥ pratyak-cetana-adhigamaḥ-api antarāya-abhāvaḥ-ca

Tatakḥ: then, from then on, starting from (the repetition). *Pratyak:* turned inwards. *Cetana:* consciousness. *Adhigamaḥ:* attainment of, achievement. *Api:* as well, even, the same. *Antarārya:* of obstacles, of hindrances. *Abhāvaḥ:* gradual absence, reduction, destruction. *Ca:* and.

I.30

The inner obstacles that disperse the mind are sickness, mental inertia, doubt, haste, apathy, intemperance, errors in judgment of oneself, lack of perseverance, and the inability to stay at a level once reached.

What are my biggest obstacles?

Can awareness of obstacles linked to my personality help me progress in yoga?

To advance further, is it necessary to overcome obstacles, find a way around them, or minimize them?

Can an obstacle serve as a means of progress?

Is finding fresh obstacles in myself already a sign of progress?

The inner obstacles presented in aphorism I.29 affect those who, lacking in active devotion, do not hear the voice from above. They can exist in any person who practices yoga.

Patañjali lists nine of them. It is possible to establish a cause-and-effect relationship between each obstacle by following the order of presentation; however, each can occur independently from the others and in no particular order. Certain obstacles crop up again and again, depending on the individuals concerned.

- Sickness (*vyādhi*) encompasses all functional disorders linked to imbalance in the constitutent elements of the body, of the driving energies, and even in the behavior.
- As a result, sickness can lead to a state of inertia or lethargy (*styāna*). The mind remains under the influence of others, or stuck in circumstances or in a lack of capacity for action.
- At this point, doubt can appear (*saṃśaya*). This is the belief that two opposing opinions are true. The beginning of the *Bhagavad Gītā* describes this state very well. The hero, *Arjuṇa,* is torn between compassion for the enemy and his duty as a warrior. It is also doubt in one's religious faith.
- Pressed by events, someone practicing yoga can be precipitated into action (*pramāda*) without reflection or concentration. An effervescence, an inattentiveness, or maladjusted and irrational behavior can bring surprising results—the opposite of those sought and even potentially dangerous, such as panic.
- The aftereffects can be total incapacity of thought and action (*ālasya*), physical and mental exhaustion, the impression of being drained of energy, after having run in all directions.
- This total lack of energy can make it quite impossible to resist the sensory, sensual, and sexual cravings that flood us (*avirati*).

- In the euphoria of pleasure, a false vision of reality can develop (*bhrāntidarśana*), an erroneous appreciation of oneself, an inferiority or superiority complex, lack of self-confidence, a defeatist attitude.
- This can sometimes explain why one cannot rise to a higher level (*alabdhabhūmikatva*), for considering one's real capacities, ambitions are without all measure.
- Or else, reaching a certain level, one falls back again (*anavasthitatvāni*), the fall being the more painful, the higher the level reached.

Such obstacles disturb the mind.

vyādhistyānasaṃśayapramādālasyāviratibhrāntidarśanālabdha-
bhūmikatvānavasthitatvāni cittavikṣepāste 'ntarāyāḥ
vyādhi-styāna-saṃaya-pramāda-ālasya-avirati-bhrānti-darśana-
alabdhabhūmikatva-anavasthitatvāni citta-vikṣepāḥ te-antarāyāḥ

Vyādhi: sickness, upset, any functional disorder. *Styāna:* inertia, mental sluggishness, lethargy. *Saṃśaya:* doubt, equivocation. *Pramāda:* effervescence, lack of concentration. *Ālasya:* apathy, indolence, laziness, mental and physical sluggishness. *Avirati:* intemperance, excessive sensuality. *Bhrāntidarśana:* slip of judgment, unjustified feeling of superiority or of inferiority. *Alabdhabhūmikatva:* incapacity to reach a new stage. *Anavasthitatvāni:* impossibility of remaining at the same level, instability. *Citta:* of spirit, of mind. *Vikṣepāḥ:* dispersion, distraction. *Te:* these, the aforesaid. *Antarāyāḥ:* obstacles.

I.31

Suffering, depression, physical restlessness, and disturbed breathing accompany mental dispersion.

Are any of these symptoms apparent in my personality?

When do they happen and with whom?

How can we estimate their real importance without minimizing, exaggerating, or misinterpreting?

What can help us observe these symptoms and see them for what they are in ourselves and others?

What is the attitude to adopt once such symptoms are recognized?

Is a psychological or psychoanalytical approach to these systems complementary or incompatible with the Yoga Sūtras?

Could all these symptoms disappear one day, or must I get used to living with them?

This aphorism introduces the symptoms connected with the obstacles listed in aphorism I.30. These range from barely perceptible to grossly visible. One or more symptoms appear to different degrees depending on the obstacle and the circumstances.

Freeing ourselves from suffering, the first symptom, is one of the basic tenets of yoga. It is often recognizing our lack of well-being that brings us to yoga. Often, we do not know the source of our suffering.

The word *duḥkha* means bad, corrupted, unclean feeling, vitiated and impure (*dus*) in the cavity (*kha*) of the heart (*hṛdayam*), the source of sensory perceptions, emotions, and sentiments. The lack of space in the heart that shadows a face and appears in bent, weary, slumped posture.

According to Vyāsa and the *Sāṃkhya-kārikāḥ* (S.K.1), such suffering is of three kinds (*duḥkhatrayam*):

- that originating in oneself (*ādhyātmikam*)
- suffering on account of others (*ādhibhautikam*)
- that arising from natural disasters (*ādhidaivikam*)

Suffering that has its source in oneself is the most accessible. Yoga addresses this kind first, defining it as something disturbing that one would like to eliminate. The *Bhagavad-Gītā* defines yoga as putting suffering at a distance (B. G.VI.23). When this kind of disturbance appears too often, it can give rise to the others.

Suffering then hits the nervous system, constantly impinging on the field of consciousness. This second symptom is depression. According to Vysa, it stems from frustration and from the fact that things hoped for do not materialize. It also stamps its mark on the face, in the attitude, and in the negative, defeatist way of speaking.

The next symptom is being unable to keep a part of the body or even the whole body still, consciously or not. This includes tics and uncontrolled movements, like the adolescent's leg that swings back and forth under the table.

The last symptom is a lack of harmony and ease with breathing. The intake, cited first, predominates. For example, unconsciously holding the breath followed by sighs.

The first two symptoms are psychological and the last two are physical. Noticing such symptoms informs us of the presence of inner obstacles, just as smoke denotes fire. It helps us to choose a suitable method of approach.

duḥkhadaurmanasyāṅgamejayatvaśvāsapraśvāsā vikṣepasahabhuvaḥ
duḥkha-daurmanasya-aṅgamejayatva-śvāsa-praśvāsāḥ vikṣepa - saha-bhuvaḥ

Duḥkha: pain, suffering, oppression. *Daurmanasya:* depression, prostration, neurasthenia. *Aṅgamejayatva:* physical agitation, trembling. *Śvāsa-praśvāsāḥ:* disturbed breathing in and out. *Vikṣepa:* cause of dispersion, distraction. *Saha-bhuvaḥ:* produced simultaneously, accompanying.

I.32

The persevering practice of a single principle keeps obstacles at a distance.

Am I tempted to do too much: too many activities, too many relationships, and so on?

How does self-knowledge encourage judicious choice (see the notes in I.22)?

How can I realize that I have searched long enough and that now is the time to choose a single aim toward mastery?

How can I discern when my attachment sends me in the wrong direction?

How can I evolve from quantity to quality in all aspects of my life: professional, emotional, and spiritual?

Patañjali has already presented two ways: persevering practice and nonattachment (I.12); and special devotion to *Īśvara* by repeating his name (I.23 to I.28). The third tool introduced here aims at diminishing obstacles. First in a series of eight (I.32 to I.39), it is both a method and a state of mind that should accompany the other seven.

The method is to stick to a single practice, method, and instructor without distraction. It is passing from multiplicity to unity, from quantity to quality. It is an ideal proposal for those who are unstable and in doubt (I.30). However, it is not advisable for those with schizoid tendencies.

The choice of the single principle must be a good one, and one should proceed methodically.

A high, general aim, such as "become more attentive to others" is judicious, but must be approached through concrete, readily accessible objectives, such as scheduled devotional activities, for example, "Buy flowers and offer them at 6 p.m."

Some commentators maintain that a single principle means God. Thus prayer is salvation.

tatpratiṣedhārthamekatattvābhyāsaḥ
tat-pratiṣedha-artham eka-tattva-abhyāsaḥ

Tat: the latter, these, *Pratiṣedha:* elimination. *Artham:* with the aim. *Eka:* of a, of one. *Tattva:* essential principle. *Abhyāsaḥ:* persevering practice.

The mind becomes quiet when it cultivates friendliness in the presence of happiness, active compassion in the presence of unhappiness, joy in the presence of virtue, and indifference toward error.

Do I tend to be jealous of those who succeed?

Can being friendly with them assuage my feelings of inferiority?

Am I unmoved by the misfortunes of others?

Can helping and sympathizing with others lift me out of my selfishness?

Am I at a loss with virtuous people? Do I try to discourage them? Can I rejoice and share in their virtue?

Do I condemn others for their mistakes or do I trail in their wake?

How can I stay neutral and see clearly?

If we are indifferent or neutral to erroneous behavior, would such behavior go without notice? What would the consequences be?

This aphorism directly addresses our relationships with others. It proves that yoga is not only for ascetics living in solitude. It points out the appropriate attitude to develop in daily life.

Faced with the four situations set out above, certain erroneous, affective impulses agitate the mind, which itself is a source of inappropriate reactions.

A negative person tends to envy a relative or a neighbor who is more successful, which aggravates his or her situation. Becoming a friend of the lucky can diminish the sadness of someone "who never has a chance."

Passing on the opposite side of the street to avoid being upset by another's unhappiness reinforces the isolation of the egocentric person. Coming to the aid of the unfortunate can open him or her to others.

We may feel our own shortcomings when we see others do the good we had not thought of ourselves, or by noticing quite simply that we are incapable of doing so. Rejoicing in another's goodness and appreciating the useful gesture can calm our minds.

When faced with evil, we can be tempted to play the part of righter of wrongs, or let ourselves be implicated in the same thing. Neutrality keeps us calm. Of course, it goes without saying that neutrality does not mean abandoning our responsibilities. But, to exercise them correctly, the mind must be calm.

Any relationship can be classed in one of the four categories listed by Patañjali in this aphorism.

Aphorism II.14 introduces the cause-and-effect relationship between the good that leads to happiness and the evil that leads to unhappiness.There is a continuity between the pairs friendship-happiness and joy-virtue on the one hand, and between compassion-unhappiness and neutrality-error on the other. Two pairs are often present together. For example, drinking provokes physical and mental pain. One can have a neutral approach to drinking and an active feeling of compassion for the sufferings of the alcoholic.

The attitudes advised here are quite the opposite of erroneous reactions. It is illusion to wish to impose them on oneself. What is proposed is analysis, which allows us to improve our reactions and responses.

In this respect we can put this aphorism alongside attitudes toward others (*yama*) or to oneself (*niyama*) presented in aphorism II.30.

maitrīkaruṇāmuditopekṣāṇāṃ sukhaduḥkhapuṇyāpuṇyaviṣayāṇāṁ bhāvanātaścittaprasādanam
maitrī-karuṇā-muditā-upekṣāṇāṃ sukha-duḥkha-puṇya-apuṇya-viṣayāṇāṃ bhāvanātaḥ-citta-prasādanam

Maitrī: friendship, love. *Karuṇā:* compassion, pity. *Muditā:* joy. *Upekṣāṇām:* neutrality, indifference; *Sukha:* happiness, (to be) at ease. *Duḥkha:* pain, suffering, oppression. *Puṇya:* good action, virtue, good, justice. *Apuṇya:* bad action, vice, evil. *Viṣayāṇām:* (with regard to) objects. *Bhāvanātaḥ:* because of the mental attitude. *Citta:* of the mind. *Prasādanam:* purification, serenity, tranquillity.

The mind also attains serenity through prolonged exhalation and holding the breath.

Does it calm the mind to recite a word or a positive phrase mentally while prolonging the exhale, then briefly pausing between breaths?

To breathe this way, does one need a certain ease or inner calm, and fullness of breath?

Can a person suffering from respiratory insufficiency breathe this way without the help of an experienced teacher?

Another way of stabilizing the mind is to be attentive to the whole process of breathing—especially breathing out and holding the breath to good purpose.

Mental processes are closely linked with the breath. An agitated mind disturbs breathing. Calming the breathing process, therefore, can quiet the mind. This has the added benefit of bringing to awareness a process that is otherwise automatic and unconscious. This opens the way to progressive changes in physiology and behavior.

The emphasis is on exhaling, by which we eliminate impurities on the physiological, psychological, and even spiritual levels. Suspending the breath after exhalation corresponds to humility and sacrifice.

Breathing is presented here, for the first time, as a way to reduce mental dispersion. It may often just be a case of sitting or lying down and becoming aware of one's breathing until one feels a greater inner calm. This mastery is acquired by practicing breath control, the development of which is described at the end of Chapter II (II.49, 50, 51).

pracchardanavidhāraṇābhyāṃ vā prāṇasya
pracchardana-vidhāraṇbhyāṃ vā prāṇasya

Pracchardana: breathing out. *Vidhāraṇābhyām:* holding the breath, apnea, control. *Vā:* or else. *Prāṇasya:* of the breath.

I.35

Objective sensory perception stabilizes and focuses thought.

Is my perception of myself and others objective?

Am I more objective in family surroundings, at work, in study, or in leisure pursuits?

Can others' remarks about me encourage me to work toward this high level of objectivity?

What attitudes are obstacles to objectivity?

What connection can we make between this high level of objectivity and judicious expression?

Our senses are doors to our environment. We should control them, yet very often they control us, enslaving us with the objects they show us. A direct way to yoga is to free ourselves from this bondage.

Objective perception of self and others prevents projection (see commentary on I.3). We face our difficulties and problems, no longer seeing them as larger than life, but as relative to everything else. Through this essential means a yoga teacher becomes more attentive to students' individual needs without imposing his or her own path or method on them.

On a concrete level, a high level of objectivity refines sensory perception: sight, hearing, taste, smell, and touch, as well as consciousness of self in relationship with another. Without doing or saying anything, by his or her simple presence alone, the observer already influences the one observed. One good method for overcoming enslavement to the senses is to verify ones attitude briefly before and after taking action. Believers can find help by turning their minds to God.

viṣayavatī vā pravṛttirutpannā manasaḥ sthitinibandhinī
viṣayavatī vā pravṛttiḥ-utpannā manasaḥ sthiti-nibandhinī

Viṣayavatī: highly objective perception. *Vā:* or else. *Pravṛttiḥ:* development. *Utpannā:* produced (by). *Manasaḥ:* of thought. *Sthiti:* stability. *Nibandhinī:* bound, linked, links, which binds.

Mental stability also stems from serenity linked to luminous lucidity.

Can I easily maintain serenity even when I'm faced with my suffering and distress?

To sustain serenity, is it better:

- *always to see the bright side and avoid seeing what is going wrong?*
- *to look clearly at what is going wrong in its relativity to everything else?*

Is it easier to be lucid if I perceive or think for myself, or if I allow a higher force to see in and through me?

Without lucidity, can the state in which perception of suffering is absent be dangerous?

Without a relative absence of perception of suffering, can lucidity be destructive?

This way of working explores a subtle universe: that of the feelings and the heart evoked by the following:

- Physical and psychological well-being and deep serenity, which diminish suffering. This way is related to contentment (*saṃtoṣa,* II.42). Such positive vision requires lucidity or insight into the self.
- Light originates in the center of the heart (*hṛdayam*) wherein is found, according to the Hindu tradition, divine presence. Some also say light originates at the top of the head (III.25 and III.32).

In this mystical, contemplative state of peace, one feels the life that animates all beings and everything in nature and establishes a deep relationship with it. To this end, yoga proposes the practice of *yoni mudrā:* Visualize divine light in the heart with eyes and ears closed, and focus the mind on the spot between the eyebrows while holding the breath, lungs full, reciting *mantras.*

The development of serenity without self-complacency leads to the yoga state.

viśokā vā jyotiṣmatī
viśokā vā jyotiṣmatī

Viśokā: serenity, absence of pain, *Vā:* or else. *Jyotiṣma-tī:* luminous, full of light (*jyotis:* spirituality, divine energy).

I.37

Turning to a being whose mind is released from passions is also calming.

In the midst of torment do I:

- *ask a calm, experienced person for help?*
- *wonder what this person would do in my position?*
- *seek the light of an inspired author?*

What is the connection between this means and the relationship of master to student?

Am I reluctant to use this means? Why?

How do these two attitudes develop:

- *devoting all my time to concentrating on my model?*
- *acting only through someone else?*

How can I choose a good model?

Does such a means recall the psychoanalytical notion of transfer?

When upset, a child turns to its mother. An adult adrift can call for help from someone freed from his or her passions. The person toward whom one turns can be near or far, living or departed. The person's writings or testimony can serve as reference. Religions hold this sort of inclination.

Maybe one can concentrate on the great peace this superior being has attained. Or perhaps one may begin to see one's way clear by reflecting on how this person might have been in a similar situation. The mind takes color from its object and can become like those it frequents.

To free ourselves from excessive passion, we can concentrate on a being free of passion. First we must redirect this passion toward a free being, a mediator. This is a delicate choice. This being must have resolved his or her own problems and be above suspicion.

vītarāgaviṣayaṃ vā cittam
vīta-rāga-viṣayaṃ vā cittam

Vita-rāga: whose passions are appeased. *Viṣayam:* taking for object (on which one places one's attention). *Vā:* or else. *Cittam:* the mind.

Mental stability also flows from the consciousness in dream and deep sleep.

Does preparing for sleep improve my attention for the next day?

Can one prepare for sleep by modifying the quantity or kinds of activities, leisure pursuits, meals, and so on?

Do I sleep too much or too little or well or badly?

Are my dreams distressing and futile or symbolic and significant?

Can I interpret them myself by meditating on their meaning?

How can I prevent this inquiry from distracting me from daily life?

According to the Vedic tradition, deep sleep (*nidrā*) (I.10) is a particular state. Though the mind is in contact with its pure source, God, it is unconscious of what is happening. We become aware of the quality of sleep only afterwards—"I've had a good sleep." The vitality one feels on waking does not come from physiological rest, but from retapping the vitalizing source of a spiritual encounter.

An inquiry on sleep and preparation for it should take the individual constitution into account (see *vāta-pitta-kapha,* aphorism I.22). A predominance of wind (*vāta*) can show itself in dreams of movement in space, falls, and chases; of bile (*pitta*), in dreams of fire and attacks; and of phlegm (*kapha*), in dreams of water, pools, and clouds. Dreaming corresponds to the imagination presented in aphorism I.9.

Once the mind is pacified, dreams well up from the deep levels of the the inner being (*draṣṭar*). It is better to meditate on a highly symbolic dream than on an unpleasant one.

An inquiry in this direction helps to stabilize thought in certain personalities attracted to all that is beyond the waking state. Above all, this study can better anchor them in daily life. Don't we say: "The night brings counsel?"

svapnanidrājñānālambanaṃ vā
svapna-nidrā-jñāna-ālambanaṃ vā

Svapna: of sleep with dreams, dream, reverie. *Nidrā:* of deep sleep (dreamless). *Jñāna:* knowledge. *Ālambanam:* support, prop, rest. *Vā:* or else.

I.39

Choosing meditation according to one's affinities also brings mental stability.

Should I choose an object with religious, visual, or aural character? Or perhaps an object with all of these qualities, for example, a visual representation of God with the repetition of God's name?

Is such a choice intuitive or rational, and can I choose without help?

In the beginning at least, is it better to choose an object that is:

- *visual (image) if one is passionate, extroverted, and active?*
- *sonorous (chant, mantra) if one is more inward and passive (I.15)?*

Is the meditation proposed here best done seated with eyes closed, or in an active state with eyes open?

This method complements the preceding ones, opening the field to every possibility. There is total freedom of choice, except for one condition: one must feel drawn to the object, especially at first. As time goes on, mastery allows the choice of varied objects. Any "object" is possible: a sound, a text, a *mantra,* a symbol, an aphorism, a mental attitude, and for believers, God.

Objects, statues, icons, and images that represent a saint or a teaching, visually or otherwise, provide a link that becomes a provisional focus for the mind. This bridge leads to what the object represents. If, in the beginning the actual presence of the object is useful, later just calling it to mind can be sufficient. Becoming excessively attached to the chosen object results only in dependence, not in meditation. The object cannot become an attachment, but at the same time, its choice must be the result of powerful motives.

Aphorism II.11 presents meditation as a means of reducing the causes of suffering. Aphorisms II.29 and III.2 present it as the seventh limb of yoga. Aphorism (IV.6) presents it as a superior means to avoid influencing others in a negative way.

yathābhimatadhyānādvā
yathā-abhimata-dhyānāt-vā

Yathā: according to, conforming with. *Abhimata:* agreeable, wished for, desired. *Dhyānāt:* (because of) meditation. *Vā:* or else.

Control of the mind then extends to the infinitely small and the infinitely vast.

Am I as at ease in great debates on ideas as I am in seeing to the small details of daily life?

Are my thoughts and my conceptual speech just made up of abstract ideas or are they concrete—based on examples?

If I am better at analyzing the slightest details, is it in my interest to develop the skill of synthesis in order to understand things as a whole?

Conversely, if I am better at synthesis, should I develop an analytic capacity?

How does mastery of the infinitely small and the infinitely vast relate to divine omniscience (I.23 to I.26)?

What about the belief that meditating on God alone widens vision to encompass God within, thus seeing each detail of nature as clearly as God does?

This aphorism presents the result of completely mastering the mind, or understanding everything that can enter the field of consciousness in its two extremes: the infinitely vast and the infinitely small.

Very often people with a good capacity for synthesis have little affinity for practical details that require an analytic capacity, and vice versa. Similarly, mystical temperaments are not always at ease in dealing with material questions and vice versa. There are those who give precedence to long-term views over the immediate, and vice versa.

paramuparamahattvānto 'sya vaśīkāraḥ
paramāṇu-parama-mahattva-antaḥ-asya vaśīkāraḥ

Paramāñu: infinitely small, an infinitesimal part. *Parama:* supreme or extreme. *Mahattva:* greatness, vastness. *Antaḥ:* limit, edge, end. *Asya:* of this latter (the mind). *Vaśīkāraḥ:* mastery, submission to the will.

I.41

As fluctuations subside, the contemplative mind becomes transparent like a gem, and reflects the object, whether it is that which perceives, the instrument of perception, or the object perceived.

A transparent gem immediately takes on the color of its surroundings without losing its purity and without retaining any trace of the previous contact. Yet, it remains resilient and solid (a diamond's hardness is well known). How can this powerful analogy help me to improve mentally and psychically?

What circumstances of my life encourage development of such transparency: professional, familial, religious, meditative, or other aspects?

Is real transparency:

- *free of color, that is, free of personal reaction? Is such a thing possible?*
- *perception of our own coloration in another without attributing it to the other?*

When emotions no longer ripple through my mind, it then reflects reality like a still water surface. How and when should I pause to let my mind settle and become transparent once more?

How can I distinguish between real contemplation and mere quiet mind?

Patañjali devotes the last part of Chapter I to describing contemplation and its different levels, but only after having set clear conditions for beginning yoga and defining it with regard to the mind, then describing the mind, several means of access to the yoga state, and obstacles and their symptoms.

Contemplation is characterized by the absence of mental fluctuation. The mind turns in one direction, undistracted. As a transparent gem faithfully reflects the color of the light, the mind reflects reality without coloring it with its individual tendency. In a state of perfect receptivity, the three elements of perception are themselves transparent.

In the first stage, the shape of a flower, for example, is the object the eye (the instrument of perception) glimpses. The eye presents the image to the mind (which perceives). If one continues to perceive, the eye itself may become the object: it distinguishes more or less clearly, it gets tired, sight may become more luminous or cloudy.

At a more subtle level, the mind becomes "that which perceives." If we push the experience further, we begin to observe sentiments—"I like or I do not like observing the flower." Then the eye becomes the object. At a level even deeper than that of mind as perceiving instrument is the superior entity—"that which perceives." In light of this superior entity, all the other levels are ephemeral, transitory, and fluctuating.

When one is able to maintain, without inhibition or will, for some time and in one direction only, a peaceful relationship among being, mind, senses, and an object, one integrates with the whole and enters contemplation.

Such an experience leads to different states depending on the object and the degree of mental purity. A mystical theme as object leads to a different experience than an exterior object as theme.

For a believer, the object (*grāhya*) represents God, the instrument (*grahaṇa*) is the mind and the senses, and the perceiving agent (*grahītṛ*) is one's inner being (see commentary in I.3).

kṣīṇavṛtterabhijātasyeva maṇergrahītgrahaṇagrāhyeṣu
tatsthatadanjañatā samāpattiḥ
kṣīṇa-vṛtte abhijātasya iva maṇeḥ grahītṛ-grahaṇa-grāhyeṣu
tat-stha-tad-añjanatā samāpattiḥ

Kṣīṇa: diminished, weakened, reduced. *Vṛtteḥ:* fluctuations, movements, activities. *Abhijātasya:* purified, of quality, transparent. *Iva:* as if, so to say. *Maṇeḥ:* the precious stone, jewel, or gem. *Grahītṛ:* in one who sees and knows. *Grahaṇa:* in the instrument of perception. *Grāhyeṣu:* in the object glimpsed, known. *Tat-stha:* being firmly set in that (the object). *Tad-añjanatā:* taking on characteristics or coloring. *Samāpattiḥ:* contemplation.

I.42

It then becomes contemplation with a mixed approach, in which representations of the object remain: its name, its essence, and the knowledge one has of it.

Can I understand my choice through my personal impressions, then recognize and go beyond personal impressions to see things correctly—to see otherwise?

How do I see my own distortions and go beyond them?

Is an external, neutral observer indispensable for that?

What can this aphorism teach me about passing on my own experience?

Aphorisms I.42 to I.44 introduce four stages of the contemplation described in the preceding aphorism.

The first stage is addressed here: Although the mind functions in one direction, the object still provokes the reaction of naming it and an experience in the emotional sphere, which partially clouds its intrinsic reality, its unique character. Experience has conditioned perception up to this point. Of necessity, we must pass these inner reference points allowing us to recognize the object. No grasp is possible without a scale of values or without experience. Accurate grasp does not exist, however, until we go further than this first stage.

Even religions that proscribe visual or verbal representation of God use texts or other supports that allow an approach of "One who is above all."

tatra śabdārthajñānavikalpaiḥ saṅkīrṇā savitarkā samāpattiḥ
tatra śabda-artha-jñāna-vikalpaiḥ saṅkīrṇā savitarkā samāpattiḥ

Tatra: there, in that place, then. *Śabda:* name, word. *Artha:* signification, essence, aim. *Jñāna:* knowledge. *Vikalpaiḥ:* imagination, ideation, representation, mental constructions. *Saṅkīrṇā:* mixed, composed of. *Savitarkā:* with analytical knowledge, deductive. *Samāpattiḥ:* contemplation.

Beyond the mixed approach stage, contemplation manifests the exact nature of the object. Memory is totally purified, as if the mind were stripped of its identity.

Am I ready to free enough physical and mental space in my life to prepare access to this stage?

How do we prepare to approach the divine without creating attachment?

Is purified memory no longer subjective, or is it that we have more or less eliminated subjectivity and become fully conscious of what remains?

How does this experience affect the personality?

In the preceding stage of contemplation, the name of the object, its intrinsic reality, and the emotional impact existed side by side. What remains is intrinsic reality alone. Past experiences, sentiments, and personal judgments no longer interfere in the relationships between the consciousness, which is witness, and the object. Such an experience appears when one holds attention long enough for the other modes of consciousness to fade out. Union with the object intensifies and one becomes immersed in it. We are no longer conscious of our own particular identity. The expression "as if" (*iva*) is important. If there is a loss of conscious reflection in that state, it reappears afterward.

In a quest for God, beatitude is indescribable, except in the case of artistic expression. God's presence is so overwhelming that no representation can fully express it. To reach such a high level, a long purification using postures, breathing, chanting, and appropriate food and way of life are indispensable. This stage approaches the powers discussed in Chapter III.

smṛtipariśuddhau svarūpaśūnyevārthamātranirbhāsā nirvitarkā

smṛti-pariśuddhau sva-rūpa-śūnyā iva artha-mātra-nirbhāsā nirvitarkā

Smṛti: memory. *Pariśuddhau:* in complete purification. *Svarūpa:* its own shape. *Śūnyā:* emptiness, lacking. *Iva:* as if. *Artha:* essence, exact nature. *Mātra:* only, nothing but. *Nirbhāsā:* manifestation, appearance, brilliance. *Nirvitarkā:* contemplation beyond analytical knowledge.

I.44

Such contemplation intuitively grasps subtle objects in their reality and beyond.

Am I more at home exploring concrete realities or metaphysical concepts?

How can I become transparent to intuitions, verify their truth by reasoning, and use them creatively?

What part do the mind and heart play in passing from a superficial level to the inner level?

Is subtlety more at the level of the object or in the individual's faculty to grasp subtlety?

The notion of "object" (*viṣayā*) is a vast one. It describes the element on which contemplation is based. Two categories can be distinguished: the physical and the metaphysical universes. Similarly, one can perceive most objects at different levels, ranging from their outer form to their very concept—their symbolic sense.

If the first two stages of contemplation (I.42 and I.43) apply more particularly to crude objects or to the rough aspects of objects, the stages of contemplation presented here allow for a relationship with subtle objects or the subtle aspects of objects.

A personal difficulty is a crude object, at least when one first explores it. Seeking to encounter God concerns the subtle level. In the fourth stage of contemplation, the individual (*dhyāta*) becomes the object (*dhyeya*). Lived-through experience transcends all logical understanding. The four stages of contemplation are successive and exploratory, because crude objects are easier to grasp and understand, and because one runs less risk of deceiving oneself about one's own realizations.

etayaiva savicārā nirvicārā ca sūkṣmaviṣayā vyākhyātā
etayā eva savicārā nirvicārā ca sūkṣma-viṣayā vyākhyātā

Etayā: by these latter. *Eva:* precisely. *Savicārā:* contemplation with a subtle grasp, correct intuition. *Nirvicārā:* contemplation beyond subtle grasp, beyond correct intuition. *Ca:* and. *Sūkṣma:* subtle. *Viṣayā:* the object of which. *Vyākhyātā:* explained.

Subtlety of the object is limitless, except that it must manifest itself.

Can knowing that self-perception is limitless encourage me to search more and more deeply?

Is it impossible to glimpse the very source of perception (apart from its manifestations) Does this limit my endeavor?

For a believer, can God only be glimpsed through manifestation?

Is there a connection between this aphorism and aphorism I.40 (control of the mind)?

This aphorism defines the limits of the mind's capacity to perceive objects. Ranging from the visible to the invisible, understanding would be limitless, attaining all, if not for the source of perception. This origin can only be glimpsed through its manifestations, even those of infinite subtlety.

The most subtle manifestation is the joy, the beatitude, the infinite love that emanates from this source and allows a correct vision of reality in and around oneself.

sūkṣmaviṣayatvaṃ cāliṅgaparyasānam
sūkṣma-viṣayatvaṃ ca aliṅga-paryavasānam

Sūkṣma: subtle. *Viṣayatvam:* being an object. *Ca:* and. *Aliṅga:* in the absence of marking, unmanifest, beyond distinctive signs. *Paryavasānam:* its final stage, finishing.

I.46

These four contemplative stages comprise contemplation with seed.

How does knowing we each bear the seed of contemplation within affect my view of myself and others?

What attitudes, what actions, what acceptance would help to germinate this seed?

What objects would help me to grow toward contemplation: abstract concepts, religious objects, inquiries on the psychological level, my everyday attitudes and actions, or any other object?

This seed within contemplation is a starting point and a support through progressive stages. Presented in its different guises in aphorisms I.42, I.43 and I.44, we can compare it with that introduced in aphorism I.17.

The choice of the word seed (*bīja*) calls to mind the following ideas:

- This seed state is in every individual.
- This seed, as aphorism IV.3 clarifies, contains within itself the necessary potential for its development.
- It is necessary to remove all obstacles to its growth by furnishing it with favorable conditions. As T.K.V. Desikachar has said, "They also involve preparation, gradual progression, and sustained interest. For without this interest, there will be distraction. Without preparation, there can be no foundation. And without gradual progression, the human system may react and rebel."*
- The development of the seed of contemplation requires an exterior object as a starting point. Beginning with the origin of the inquiry, understanding gradually becomes clearer until it becomes total. Grasp of the object implies a good grasp of oneself focused on the object.

Only where there is reality and patience can there be contemplation.

tā eva sabja samdhi
tāḥ eva sabja samdhi

Tāḥ: these, the latter (states of contemplation). *Eva:* precisely, exactly. *Sabījaḥ:* with the seed, source, origin. *Samādhiḥ:* contemplation.

With the mastery of the fourth seed of contemplation, the inner being appears in all clarity and serenity.

Am I ready to accept the mirror that others offer me?

How can serenity help me tackle the problem of lucidity about myself?

How can a believer prepare to receive the grace that leads to a correct view of personality, of deeper nature, and of the presence of God within?

How do lucidity and serenity affect my activities and relationships, both with myself and with others?

This aphorism describes the results of the fourth seed of contemplation, which transcends all attachment—even attachment to the finest of perceptions. It is then possible to be conscious of true reality instantaneously, regardless of circumstances. In a way, it is like the quotation attributed to Socrates, "Know thyself and thou shalt know the universe." Such lucidity about oneself corresponds to a state of inner peace, as if any superfluous movement of the mind were an obstacle to perception.

For a believer, this aphorism corresponds to awareness of the radiant divine presence in oneself. Someone who reaches this high level of peace and insight may be compared to a climber on an alpine summit. He or she sees everything in a twinkling and understands just where the other alpine climbers stand in their progress toward the summit. The mystery of life becomes clear.

Entering into contemplation with "external" objects, one not only discovers their essence, but also one's own.

nirvicāravaiśāradye 'dhyātmaprasādaḥ
nirvicāra-vaiśāradye-adhyātma-prasādaḥ

Nirvicāra: of contemplation over and above correct intuition. *Vaiśāradye:* in maturity, expert. *Adhyātma:* of the supreme being, spiritual. *Prasādaḥ* serenity, clarity, illumination.

I.48

Now the outflowing of supreme knowledge is absolute truth.

If it is true that everyone has their own form of truth, does perceiving absolute truth mean that:

- *I accept all points of view?*
- *I realize the limits of my own truth?*
- *I never again make mistakes?*
- *I instantly recognize my mistakes?*

Can we encompass the totality of this absolute truth or can we only glimpse part of it?

Once we cleanse and pacify the mind, knowledge is no longer unconsciously tainted by affective impulses, sentiments, or innate or acquired personal tendencies. We directly and instantaneously grasp reality as it is. Messages transmitted by the sense organs correspond to the reality of the objects themselves, and actions are adapted to each circumstance.

Doubt is absent, vision is pure, words irrefutable, and actions correct.

Qualifying this supreme knowledge as bearer of supreme truth (*ṛtaṁ bharā*) indicates that it is real wisdom (*prajñā*). The flawless (*satyam* II.36) words and actions of the sage are eternal.

ṛtaṃbharā tatra prajñā
ṛtaṃ-bharā tatra prajñā

Ṛtam: the highest truth, justice, religious law. *Bharā:* bearer of. *Tatra:* there, in that place, at that moment. *Prajñā:* the highest knowledge.

This supreme knowledge grasps the intrinsic nature of the object, which differs from the correct knowledge that tradition and inference bring.

Why do I seek answers and solutions in the traditions or in a personal effort of analysis?

What qualities can help me wait, a long time if necessary, for a direct intuitive grasp to flash through my mind?

Is direct and instantaneous higher grasp useful primarily for certain categories of objects? If so, what are they?

How have tradition and inference enabled me to attain an intuitive grasp that transcends them?

Two modes of grasping reality are opposed in this aphorism. Dependent on the mind and its mistakes, the lower level presents reality in two ways:

- through tradition—the teachings of the sacred writings, the instructions, and the testimonies that guide us, whether these issue from living witnesses or not
- through inference, which represents logical research and analysis

Neither of these two approaches allows perfect grasp of the intrinsic reality of the object.

Only knowledge that issues from contemplation and transcends the verbal or analytic grasp allows this. The mind, perfectly transparent, no longer gets in the way. Perception is instantaneous. The believer sees in it submission to the Lord.

Yoga, therefore, emphasizes the direct relationship with the object of contemplation, unlike other systems of traditional *Vedic* thought.

śrutānumānaprajñābhyāmanyaviṣayā viśeṣārthatvāt
śruta-anumāna-prajñābhyām anya-viṣayā viśeṣa-arthatvtā

Śruta: heard, understood, testimony, tradition, revelation from a master. *Anumāna:* inference, induction, deduction. *Prajñābhyām:* (of two) correct forms of knowledge. *Anya:* different, other. *Viṣayā:* coming from an object. *Viśeṣa:* specificity, particularity with a sense of superiority. *Arthatvāt:* (from its ability to grasp) the very nature (of), intrinsic reality.

I.50

Mental permeation born of direct knowledge opposes all other mental permeation.

Do I change my habits often or do I hedge myself in with conditioning?

How can I develop the habit of taking time for silence, so I can hear the inner reply?

Am I resisting this change?

What daily routine might encourage this new habit?

What influence does this new mental conditioning have on my relationships with others?

The expression "mental permeation" (I.18) represents an essential mode of human functioning. Our behavior is conditioned by the past. The greater the attention we pay to an act, the greater its influence on future action. The influence takes concrete form in a series of habitual behaviors that are often unconscious.

Yoga differentiates between two kinds of mental permeation. The first results from agitated thought and unpurified emotion. The second results from a deep-seated state of mental peace and compassion—the state of contemplation. This second kind of permeation opposes returning to the previous one. It would be an illusion to try to live without any habits at all. It is preferable to replace negative conditioning little by little with positive attitudes, including, in spite of the paradox, the one condition of being free. Then spontaneity flows and thoughts and actions are instantaneous and correct. Being in the present moment is total. The habit of such spontaneity prevents the reappearance of thought based on memory and reasoning. Always thinking about things becomes tiring. Remaining available, present, and open enables one to see clearly—immediately.

tajjaḥ saṃskāro 'nyasaṃskārapratibandhī
tad-jaḥ saṃskāraḥ-anya-saṃskāra-pratibandhī

Tad: this, the latter (direct knowledge). *Jaḥ:* born of, engendered by. *Saṃskāraḥ:* mental permeation resulting from past acts. *Anya:* other. *Saṃskāra:* mental permeation. *Pratibandhī:* opposes.

In passing beyond this last kind of mental permeation, seedless contemplation appears.

Does ending all mental permeation mean that our habits or rituals disappear, or does it mean we can respect them in our freedom?

How can I free myself from all conditioning, but still respect the conditioning others need?

Does this require a lot of time and patience? How can I develop this?

How do I attain seedless contemplation and still lead a life with family and profession? Am I ready to meet the right guide for that?

The first chapter ends as it began (I.2), with the concept of cessation or control (*nirodaḥ*). If yoga ends fluctuations of mind by focusing on the mind's functions, even transparency must be left behind.

Seedless contemplation, a state of total spontaneity, above all desire—even the desire to know—is related to another kind of contemplation (*anyaḥ*) (I.18). It is the natural state for predestined beings (*videha* and *prakṛtilayānām,* I.19) and the state of ultimate serenity (*kaivalya*). (*see Chapter IV*).

Aphorism (I.50) alludes twice to conditioning. The notion of cessation opposes this. In the states of contemplation with a seed, positive permeations oppose negative ones. Seedless contemplation, however, is beyond all permeation. According to T.K.V. Desikachar,* "The mind reaches a state when it has no impressions of any kind. It is open, clear, simply transparent."

This is the yoga state. One cannot will it, nor receive it verbally. The pure consciousness of the inner being alone shines there (I.3).

ॐ ॐ ॐ

tasyāpi nirodhe sarvanirodhānnirbījaḥ samādhiḥ
tasya api nirodhe sarva-nirodhāt nirbījaḥ samādhiḥ

Tasya: of this, this latter (contemplation with seed). *Api:* as well, even, again. *Nirodhāt:* in the cessation, control. *Sarva:* of all (mental permeation). *Nirodhāt:* from cessation, control. *Nirbjīaḥ:* seedless. *Samādhiḥ:* contemplation.

*Patañjali's *Yogasūtras*: An Introduction, Translation and commentary by T.K.V. Desikachar (Affiliated East-West Press P. Ltd.)

CHAPTER II

METHOD

sadhānapādaḥ

METHOD

In this chapter, Patañjali describes the goal—contemplation. He then describes the way of realizing it, method, which addresses personal problems that are likely to arise.

Am I ready to acknowledge my problems and use this awareness in a positive way to overcome them?

What can I learn from Patañjali's approach of learning about the goal before learning the method to achieve it?

Can this approach help me overcome difficulties?

When studying the pathology of the human psyche, how can I keep from imagining that I have all the symptoms?

The five personality types of aphorism I.1 may be more simply differentiated into two main categories:

- Those whose minds are stable: These people are rare and can attain yoga using the very difficult, mental approach set out in Chapter I.
- Those who are absent-minded: These people attain their goal by following the yoga of action, which addresses the difficulties of active life, and the yoga of the eight limbs, which covers all levels of human life, as set out in Chapter II.

The aphorisms in Chapter II answer the following questions:

II.1 and 2	What is the yoga of action?
II.3 to 16	What obstacles do our personalities present?
II.17 to 27	What are the two levels of being?
II.28 to 55	How do the eight limbs help me to attain the yoga state?

sādhanapādaḥ
sādhana-pādaḥ

Sādhana: accomplishment, means, method, instrument, cause.
Pādaḥ: chapter, foot, quarter.

II.1

The yoga of action is a way of discipline involving self-reflection based on the sacred texts, and surrendering the fruits of action to a higher force.

Does my yoga practice enhance my involvement in daily life?

Am I more suited to the support offered by physical discipline, self-reflection, or surrender?

Do I use these three supports to enhance my practice? Am I lackadaisical about some or extreme about others?

What could happen if these three supports are unbalanced?

Does one support give rise to the others?

Can we be self-disciplined and still not discover who we are? Can we discover who we are without perceiving something higher than ourselves?

If my daily life does not improve from my practice of yoga, how can this aphorism help me?

Is there a connection between inner freedom and surrendering the fruits of action to a higher force?

In an era that emphasizes an active life, in which work has become the principal measure of human value and society is materialistic, yoga must be a yoga of action. Spiritual evolution must be tested in active engagement.

The yoga of action is a way of evolving useful to those who are engaged in active life. A purely *Vedic* approach, this yoga stands apart from other methods that include delicate energetic practices which might prove dangerous. The yoga of action involves three disciplines, or supports, spoken of in order of their subtlety.

- The first support is the discipline of caring for ourselves physically (*tapas*). We must:
  - Purify ourselves (*tap:* heat, cook) by eliminating negative factors preventing good physical, mental, and emotional health
  - Practice yoga postures and breath control daily
  - Use moderate exercise to eliminate tensions
  - Follow a diet that is moderate and light on the digestion (sattva), neither too stimulating (*rajas*), nor too heavy (*tamas*)
- The second support, self-reflection (*svādhyāya*), is the study of sacred texts, best practiced through chanting and reciting them. If this is not possible, one may read or even listen to them. These texts are mirrors intended to enhance lucidity about

oneself and one's acts. For a yoga adept, the *Yoga-sūtras* becomes a text of reference.

- The third support, surrender and devotion (*Īśvara-praṇudhāna*), is a search for excellence in action, through which we surrender the results to a higher power.

For the believer, faith and devotion to God nourish our being (*varśva narāgni*), light up our thoughts (*jñanāgni*), and illuminate our consciousness (*daharāgni*).

Growth and evolution depend on a fine balance among the three supports of the yoga of action. The first two, discipline and self-reflection, can be learned; however, the third support, surrender, is a result.

We discover them more or less chronologically. Our first steps, often on the level of physical practice (for example, postures and breath [*tapas*]), lead us to explore the texts, which throw light on the self (*svadhyāya*). Then, an inner presence develops from which flows respectful attitude (*Īśvara-praṇidhāna*).

tapaḥsvādhyāyeśvarapraṇidhānāni kriyāyogaḥ
tapaḥ-svādhyāya-īśvara-praṇidhānāni kriyā-yogaḥ

Tapaḥ: heat, ardor, fervor, discipline, penitence. *Svādhyāya*: study, reflection on oneself, study of sacred texts, chanting. *Īśvara-praṇidhānani:* devotion to the Lord, the mental attitude of acceptance, detachment from results of action. *Kriyā*: action, realization, activity, the religious act. *Yogaḥ*: yoga.

II.2

The intent is to gradually attain contemplation and diminish the causes of suffering.

Can regular yoga practice improve my concentration and curtail my negative behavior?

If not, should I reconsider my approach, my practice, and my relationship with my teacher?

Do I habitually consider only the positive results of an action before taking stock of all the preexisting circumstances?

What is the significance of diminishing, rather than completely eliminating, the causes of suffering?

What guideposts along the way can help me to realize these two objectives?

This aphorism presents two results (*phalas*) of the yoga of action that are complementary and indissolubly linked. The intent to reduce the causes of suffering is both a starting point and a process. We gradually attain the state of contemplation, as we develop a better quality of concentration.

What links these objectives is realizing that concentration is impossible unless we reduce our personal problems and suffering. Patañjali first espouses the highest aim—contemplation—before touching on the subtler aspects of personal suffering.

The expression "causes of suffering" was first mentioned in aphorism I.24. It represents a fundamental aspect of yoga, that of casting light on human psychology by analyzing the erroneous impulses that lead to pain.

samādhibhāvanārthaḥ kleśatanūkaraṇārthaśca.
samādhi-bhāvana-arthaḥ kleśa-tanū-karaṇa-arthaḥ-ca.

Samādhi: contemplation. *Bhāvana:* to make appear, to manifest, to establish. *Arthaḥ*: intent, goal, motive, object. *Kleśa:* cause of suffering, torment, affliction. *Tanū:* tenuous, thin, slight, fine. *Karaṇa:* production, accomplishment, act. *Arthaḥ:* goal. *Ca:* and.

The causes of suffering are ignorance, consciousness of "I" (egoism), attachment, repulsion, and fear.

Does ignorance, the ego, attachment, repulsion, or fear dominate me?

Which negative impulses condition my behavior?

How are the five causes of suffering related? For example, how are the ego and fear related, or attachment and repulsion?

Can I best discover the causes of my suffering by listening to the remarks of others, by analyzing my own failures, or through the mirror of a guide?

How do these causes of suffering differ from the inner obstacles presented in aphorism I.30?

How do ignorance (II.3) and error (I.6) differ?

Is detailed observation and analysis of the causes of suffering the best way to reduce them?

Vyāsa attributes the sources of suffering to self, others, and natural catastrophes (see the commentary in I.31). The suffering that comes from oneself, as addressed in this aphorism, is the only cause of suffering on which we can take direct action. The five causes of self-induced suffering are presented below, from the most subtle to the most visible.

- Ignorance is the belief that one knows, being all the while in error. It shows itself, for example, in oft-heard remarks preceded by "I know…" or by defending one's point of view without being sure one is right.
- Consciousness of "I," presented in aphorism I.17 in a positive way as an element of contemplation, can become a source of problems when hypertrophied through an error of appreciation. The ego—"me, myself, and I"—isolates us from others, instead of being the proof of our right relations with others.
- Deep interest can become blind attachment.
- A justifiable, defensive reaction can become excessive repulsion and even aggression when taken to an extreme.
- Fear, which protects us in cases of real danger, can destroy us when it becomes inappropriate.

The last four represent excessive or inappropriate manifestations of natural impulses that become distorted and become sources of conflict. Each of these natural impulses, good in itself, becomes a poison when manifested in excess, at the wrong moment, or when mistaking the object.

Conquering one's greatest fears often enhances one's evolution. One learns to explore the world and multiply experiences without aggression, to acquire necessary belongings without becoming attached to them and, lastly, to affirm oneself in all circumstances without abusing anyone.

avidyāsmitārāgadveṣābhiniveśāḥ kleśāḥ
avidyā-asmitā-rāga-dveṣa-abhiniveśāḥ kleśāḥ

Avidyā: ignorance, misunderstanding, inexperience, erroneous certitude. Asmitā: consciousness of "I", awareness of one's existence, egoism, the ego. *Rāga:* passion, passionate desire, ardent burning interest, attachment. *Dveṣa:* repulsion, aversion, hate, hostility, antipathy. *Abhiniveśāḥ:* fear, sentiment of insecurity, stubborness in keeping alive. *Kleśāḥ:* the causes of suffering, torments, afflictions.

Ignorance is the source of the other four causes of suffering, whether these are latent, feeble, intermittent, or intense.

What is the difference between what I think I am and what I really am?

How can I begin to close this gap?

Must I manifest an impulse to be sure it is under control?

What circumstances lead to ego, attachment, repulsion, or fear?

Why is ignorance the source of the other causes of suffering and not the other way around?

Ignorance, by definition, remains hidden; however, it elicits four other causes of suffering that are always present in varying degrees of intensity:

- In the latent or slumbering state, the causes of suffering don't condition the individual, but they can spring to life again.
- If feeble, they don't disturb the individual to any grave extent.
- In the intermittent state, they may alternate with each other, or show themselves temporarily.
- In an intense state, they strongly color behavior.

Certain people are enmeshed in causes of suffering. Their path to yoga is a long one. Most people are itermittently under the influence of these impulses, and suffering arises when conditions predispose to it. People nearer the yoga state have innate or acquired mastery over these impulses. To be free and unconditioned by factors of suffering is one of yoga's intents and a sign of favorable evolution.

avidyā kṣetramuttareṣāṃ prasuptatanuvicchinnodārāṇām
avidyā kṣetram-uttareṣām prasupta-tanu-vicchinna-udārāṇām

Avidyā: ignorance, false certitude. *Kṣetram:* ground, soil, field. *Uttareṣām:* following, next, future, other. *Prasupta:* asleep, latent, inactive. *Tanu:* reduced, feeble. *Vicchinna:* intermittent, interrupted. *Udārāṇām:* active, abundant, manifested.

II.5

Ignorance is the confusion of the temporary with the permanent, the pure with the impure, anguish with the pleasure of being, and the relative with the absolute.

Am I able to see my way, more or less clearly, through any of the four domains of ignorance?

How do I:

- *avoid treating material goods as though they are permanent, yet not neglect their upkeep?*
- *recognize lack of clarity in some of my thoughts, yet remain self-confident?*
- *sustain conviviality and deep feelings without getting caught up in outer pleasures that would imprison me?*
- *always maintain openness and questioning, yet still be humble in the face of the absolute ?*

Does confusion on one level bring confusion on all levels?

Do we ever have the right to impose our own values?

Are we born with misconceptions?

Ignorance distorts actions at the the physical level, which includes thought and sentiment, and also at the spiritual level.

- On the physical level, ignorance confuses what is perishable (body, youth, material goods) with the eternal.
- On the level of thought, ignorance leads to lack of discernment; for example, thinking a thought is correct when it is not.
- On the level of sentiment, ignorance leads us to find pleasure in what can only lead to suffering; for example, with addictive substances such as drugs and alcohol.
- Lastly, on the spiritual level, ignorance can lead to mistaken beliefs about oneself. For example, we may believe we have reached a certain spiritual level or know our own reality when we are still in the preliminary stages.

Confusion can also show itself in the other direction; for example, mistaking what is eternal for something perishable.

These levels are not really separate from each other, they interact constantly. Becoming conscious of the transitory nature of the body, therefore, can put the pangs of existence in a different light.

Depending on the individual, the time of life, and thresholds of perception, our values normally evolve toward a more judicious recognition of the deep reality of the self and of all things, and, therefore, toward reducing misconception.

anityāśuciduḥkhānātmasu nityaśucisukhātmakhyātiravidyā
anitya-aśuci-duḥkha-anātmasu-nitya-śuci-sukha-ātma-
khyātiḥ-avidyā

Anitya: transitory, ephemeral, fleeting, temporary, perishable. *Aśuci:* impure, not purified. *Duḥkha:* pain, grief, distress, unhappiness. *Anātmasu:* in the nonabsolute. *Nitya:* eternal, permanent, perpetual, constant, indestructible. *Śuci:* pure, clear, and immaculate. *Sukha:* pleasure, agreeableness, happiness, ease. *Ātma:* the absolute. *Khyātiḥ:* giving a name to. *Avidyā:* ignorance.

II.6

Individual ego consciousness of "I" sees mental and physical activity as the source of consciousness.

Do I:

- *talk more than I listen?*
- *communicate better when I am in the higher position?*
- *always try to attract others' attention?*

Am I able to recognize my mistakes, accept my failures, and question myself?

Do I remain healthy around people who are sick, or the contrary?

Am I very attached to my independence and my autonomy?

Why does the word asmita mean both suffering (II.6) and contemplation (I.17)? How can I tell the difference?

Does self-knowledge help me avoid pride?

The yoga system presents a dualist philosophy that distinguishes in the individual:

- a spiritual principle, or entity, *dṛg* (the one who perceives), which is synonymous with *puruṣa* (I.16), or the source of consciousness;
- the material aspect, or the instrument of perception, *darśana* (see commentary in I.16 on the distinction between mind and matter), synonymous with *prakṛti,* or mental and psychic activity as a whole.

By choosing the verb (*dṛś*), Patañjali emphasizes the function, rather than the being, of *"the one who perceives"* (the spiritual entity present in each individual). The use of two words (*dṛg* and *darśana*) with the same root stresses the link between these two levels of being: nothing is perceived without a perceiver, nor can one perceive without there being a perceived object.

Each of these aspects in a human being represents a distinct force. These two forces are allied in a way that maintains life and development in human beings. We often live cut off from the principle of consciousness that shows itself through the physical level. According to yoga, however, it is impossible to conceive of a human being without the complementary presence of these two levels.

When we are awake, mental and psychic activity, sensory perceptions, bodily sensations and ideas, thoughts, cares, and, of course, confusion submerge higher consciousness. The fluctuating lower consciousness that feels pleasure and suffering disappears during deep sleep. The higher consciouness of which we are unconscious is then pure, in spite of our worries. When we wake up, individual consciousness takes over again, coloring the higher consciousness as it reunites with the mental, psychic, and physical instrument..

dṛgdarśanaśaktyorekātmatevāsmitā
dṛg-darśana-śaktyoḥ-eka-ātmatā-iva-asmitā

Dṛg: one who perceives, sees, observes, discerns. *Darśana:* the instrument of perception, vision, observation, discernment. *Śaktyoḥ:* of double force, capacity, faculty. *Eka:* one, a single. *Ātmatā:* essence, nature, principle. *Iva:* as if, in the same way as. *Asmitā:* consciousness of "I", awareness of one's existence, egoism, ego.

II.7

Attachment is the consequence of pleasure.

Am I passionate and attached, or am I detached?

Am I attracted more to material possessions; to intellectual, literary, and artistic riches; or to spiritual values?

Am I attached to memories and objects from my past?

To detach myself from something, is it better not to satisfy the desire, detach from the object gradually, or detach from it once and for all?

What does this aphorism say about nonattachment (I.12) and concentration on a being who is free from all passion (I.37)?

It is in the nature of pleasure to want to renew it. When desire progressively invades the mind and leads it to take action, it becomes a source of conflict and difficulty: sickness, broken relationships, encumbrance of objects, and useless possessions.

Such attachment shows itself not only with regard to material possessions (food, sex, honors, power, drugs, alcohol, tobacco, and so on), but to spiritual ones as well (tossing aside responsibilities and taking refuge in badly interpreted spiritual values, or excessive attachment to the spiritual endeavor in question).

Interest, even powerful interest, is positive, since nothing can be done where there is no interest. Passion in excess, however, is one of the principal causes of a human being's slavery. Addictions (*kleśa*) are distortions of natural functions.

sukhānuśayī rāgaḥ
sukha-anuśayī rāgaḥ

Sukha: pleasure, happiness, ease, agreeableness. *Anuśayī:* that which follows or comes after. *Rāgaḥ:* passion, passionate desire, ardent interest, attachment.

Aversion is the consequence of displeasure.

Do I have a lot of negative thoughts?

Do I tend to blame others?

Do I often start my sentences with "No…"?

What attitude should I take toward my dislikes and those of others?

Do my feelings of excessive attachment and repulsion stem more from myself or from sociocultural conditioning?

Do my attractions or aversions to situations or people change based on whether they are familiar or not?

Is masochism related to passion or repulsion?

Does repulsion happen because of, or in spite of, past actions?

Can passion exist without repulsion and vice versa? What connects them?

What is the connection between this aphorism and the means proposed in aphorism I.33?

Repulsion, or aversion, is based on past experience and the mental permeation that follows it. Whether conscious or not, it remains sealed in the memory, taking no account of the way the situation has evolved.

Resulting from the same mechanism as attachment (II.7), though its opposite, aversion may lead one to isolation or conflict. It is an active negative attitude of rejection and is one of the chief causes of failure in family, professional, and personal relationships.

duḥkhanuśayī dveṣaḥ
duḥkha-anuśayī dveṣaḥ

Duḥkha: pain, unhappiness, sadness, distress. *Anuśayī:* that which follows or comes after. *Dveṣaḥ:* repulsion, aversion, hatred, hostility, antipathy.

II.9

Fear is present even for the sage and develops from its own inherent source.

How aware am I of my fears and phobias?

Do my fears inhibit me, or do they make me behave irrationally, which increases risk?

What part does the imagination play in fear?

Should I conquer all my fears?

Does developing knowledge diminish fear?

Can consciousness of one's own worth lessen fear?

Can the ego hide fear?

Does fear change with age and in different periods of one's life?

Is there a hierarchical order to fearing neediness, fearing what others think, and fearing death?

Pleasure (II.7) and displeasure (II.8) are provoked by the external elements of repulsion or attraction. Fear, however, is inherent in a human being, even though it also has acquired elements. We are not talking only about physical fear but about existential fear as well. Existential fear amplifies and distorts the natural instinct for self-preservation. Every living organism has this fear, from the most elementary form of life to the greatest sage.

We can say that fear of the unknown develops from our attachments. It might arise if we are threatened by changes in our personality or public image, or changes in body, health, emotional relationships, or material possessions.

svarasavāhī viduṣo 'pi samārūḍho 'bhiniveśaḥ
svarasavāhī viduṣaḥ-api samārūḍhaḥ-abhiniveśaḥ

Sva: one's own. *Rasa:* sap, bone marrow, inner substance, quintessence, origin, regeneration. *Vāhī:* that which bears or carries. *Viduṣaḥ:* the sage, one who knows, who possesses knowledge. *Api:* even, same. *Samārūḍhaḥ:* that which has developed or firmly taken root. *Abhiniveśaḥ:* fear, feeling of insecurity, stubborn will (to keep oneself alive).

Recognizing inherent impulses eliminates the causes of suffering at a subtle level.

Am I calm and stable enough to use this means regularly?

Are there times when this would be more effective; for example, after yoga practice or after a period of rest, such as a vacation?

What positive thoughts and sentiments can keep me from having negative thoughts?

Should I count on others, myself, or both to reestablish equilibrium?

How can I use the proposed method without inhibiting myself?

Having presented the causes of suffering, Patañjali now proposes two ways of reducing them. His first advice works with impulses that are latent, or just about to appear. It is a matter of "putting out a fire at its inception with a glass of water. A few minutes later, a ton of water would prove insufficient."

This way uses positive thought and "thinking twice before we act" to attain mental peace, in which the mind is without movement. This is possible only if one is calm enough to sense fear when it first shows itself and recognize an attitude of attachment or opposition before it gives rise to an influx of unending thoughts. If that fails, one has to turn to the second method for help (II.11).

This aphorism warns us not to neglect the causes of suffering simply because they remain latent. They may still be reactivated, even in this state—"The better I feel, the more watchful I am."

te pratiprasavaheyāḥ sukṣmāḥ
te pratiprasava-heyāḥ sukṣmāḥ

Te: these, these latter (referring here to the five causes of suffering laid down in the preceding aphorisms). *Pratiprasava:* ceasing to produce, to produce or cultivate a countermovement. *Heyāḥ:* what one must leave behind, abandon, avoid. *Sukṣmāḥ:* subtle, fine, feeble, insignificant.

II.11

Meditation eliminates mental fluctuations set in motion by erroneous impulses.

Can I shake off obsessive thoughts by turning my attention to other things?

What object of meditation would help me develop a more balanced view of things?

When should I ask for help and from whom?

To eliminate my difficulties, is it necessary to meditate on them, or is it better to forget them?

What qualities support self-reflection?

Is a dash of humor about oneself a good beginning?

How do I progress from meditating on a given difficulty to cultivating its opposite state?

According to T. Krishnamacharya, mental disturbances fall into six classes:

- desires of the passions (*kāma*)
- anger (*krodha*)
- consuming eagerness and greed, impatience (*lobha*)
- aberration, illusion, wandering (*moha*)
- egotistical pleasure (*moda*)
- and envy or jealousy (*mātsarya*)

This aphorism offers a second method to use when these disturbances invade our thoughts and actions—meditation (first presented in aphorism I.39). Here it means using a form of mental activity to detach oneself from the subject of disturbance. It may consist of:

- diversion; for example, turning one's attention toward another object or activity, such as going away for a few days.
- reconsideration; for example, through detachment or discussion with a teacher.
- an appeal to a higher or divine force through prayer and silence.

The mind thus recovers its transparency once more.

dhyānaheyāstadvṛttayaḥ
dhyāna-heyāḥ-tad-vṛttayaḥ

Dhyāna: meditation. *Heyāḥ:* that which must be left, given up, avoided. *Tad:* these latter (designates the five causes of suffering). *Vṛttayaḥ:* fluctuations of the mind, the activities of the mind.

Acts stemming from mental disturbance leave imprints that always show themselves in some form or other, visible or invisible.

Do my thoughts, words, and actions arise from fear, repulsion, attachment, or egocentrism?

In this case, what is to be done?

Does this functioning of the psyche:

- *give rise to a sense of responsibility or lead to irresponsibility?*
- *give rise to a guilt complex?*
- *give rise to discouragement?*

Is an experience always determined or influenced by what has gone before.

This aphorism refers to the continuous chain of cause and effect that links erroneous impulses, negative actions, and their traces left in the psyche.

When mental disturbances (kleṣa) cause our actions they produce effects that themselves produce other effects. This mechanism is unavoidable, whether we are conscious of it or not and whether these effects are immediate or sometime in the future. A conditioned and historical way of reacting is handed down from generation to generation through atavism, heredity, and imitation. The infinite chain of causality stops when we act in a way that is pure, thoughtful, and not engendered by suffering.

kleśamūlaḥ karmāśayo dṛṣṭādṛṣṭajanmavedanīyah
kleśa-mūlaḥ karma-āśayaḥ dṛṣṭa-adṛṣṭa-janma-vedanīyaḥ

Kleśa: cause of suffering, torment, affliction. *Mūlaḥ:* root, base, foundation, origin, cause. *Karma:* action (the fact of doing) and the act (the result). *Āśayaḥ:* the drops of the mind, latent impression. *Dṛṣṭa janma:* birth, origin, existence as seen in the present, fully conscious, in this present life. *Adṛṣṭa janma:* unseen, in the future, without a glimmer of consciousness, in a future life. *Vedanīyaḥ:* (is) experiences discovered, uncovered, and revealed.

II.13

When these causes engender acts, their effects influence existence, time, and the experience of events.

Before I act, should I consider how my action might influence:

- *the level and quality of my existence?*
- *my perception and how I spend my time?*
- *pleasure in my daily life?*

Does such analysis serve for fleeting events as well as for choices that affect my whole life?

In working to reduce suffering, am I better suited to analyzing its origins (II.12) or its consequences (II.13)?

The preceding aphorism introduced a tool for analyzing the causes of our actions. This aphorism offers an instrument for analyzing their consequences. Using both methods helps us to become aware, to assume responsibilities, and to improve attitudes and personality. As long as thoughts and actions are rooted in disturbances, three kinds of conditioning are imposed:

- the form of our existence—our nature and social and cultural behavior, which reflects our values
- time—both the subjective perception of passing time, and the objectively measurable duration of an experience
- pleasure or the lack of it—the way we experience events

Such a tool allows us to analyze events by observing them as we live them. Afterward, it is possible to anticipate and thus avoid certain pitfalls that pertain to our personality.

sati mūle tadvipāko jātyāyurbhogāḥ
sati mūle tad-vipākaḥ jāti-āyuḥ-bhogāḥ

Sati: being (verb). *Mūle:* root, foundation, origin, cause. *Tad:* this, this latter (here mūla, root). *Vipākaḥ:* fruit, fructification, ripening, result, consequence. *Jāti:* caste, behavior, model, rank, level. *Āyuḥ:* length, duration, longevity. *Bhogāḥ:* final result, enjoyment, experience.

The three kinds of conditioning produce pleasure if the origin is positive, and torment if it is disturbed.

Do I create my own happiness, as well as my own unhappiness?

Can suppressing bad intentions and encouraging good intentions improve my life?

Can this aphorism induce me to stop complaining?

Why do pleasures shackle us as much as torments?

What role do predetermination and free will play in our actions?

Does feeling increasingly responsible for my reactions create more difficulty, or does it help me to make progress?

In looking at the three kinds of conditioning (II.13), two categories are distinguised:

- A well-founded act produces a positive experience. An act performed in good will but undertaken without lucidity, however, can mask lack of judgment and lead to pleasures that foster dependence.
- An inappropriate or ill-considered intention leads to suffering.

Patañjali thus directly links our intentions, our actions, and our well-being. He once more questions our natural tendency to think that unhappiness comes from others and suggests we be very careful about our real motives in the present, for they condition our future.

te hlādaparitāpaphalāḥ punyāpuṇyahetutvāt
te hlāda-paritāpa-phalāḥ puṇya-apuṇya-hetutvāt

Te: these (latter) (designates *jāti, āyu,* and *bhoga,* the three types of result seen in the preceding aphorism). *Hlāda:* joy. *Paritāpa:* the burn, anguish, torment, remorse. *Phalāḥ:* fruit, effect, result. *Puṇya:* just, correct, adequate, appropriate, proper, virtuous, virtue. *Apuṇya:* incorrect, inadequate, inappropriate, improper, vicious, vice. *Hetutvāt:* the fact of being at the origin, of a cause.

II.15

The discerning person sees that all is suffering, because of changes due to the passage of time, to worries and conditioning, and to inappropriate manifestations of the constituent qualities of nature.

Seeing that my thoughts, words, and actions can cause suffering, am I watchful enough?

Am I most vulnerable to time-related changes (pariṇāmas), to worries and conditioning, (saṃskāras), or to dependency on desires (tāpas) such as tobacco and alcohol?

Am I dominated by inertia or overactivity, or do I alternate between the two?

How do I simultaneously develop discernment (in order to become aware that all is potential suffering), and serenity (I.36)?

Is awareness of the possible deep suffering of each being dangerous, progressive, or advantageous?

Is this aphorism optimistic, pessimistic, or realistic?

This aphorism asserts that as we become more discerning we see suffering everywhere. Though we may see this as negative and pessimistic, the discerning person acknowledges suffering. He or she perceives that immediate pleasure can also be a source of suffering.

There are two possible sources of suffering. One is the interplay between the human psyche and its surroundings, examples of which are:

- changes brought about by time and old age
- ills, pangs, and unrealizable, inappropriate desires and whims
- rigidity created by one's own mental and cultural constructions

All of these factors lead to suffering, either separately or because they come into conflict, especially in the form of conflicting habits (*saṃskāra*) and because of the inevitable passage of time (*pariṇāma*). Certain personalities adapt better to change, whereas others need habits and routine (see *Āyurveda* typology in aphorism I.22).

The second source of suffering comes from the different colorations in the psyche created by the incessant changes in the constituent qualities of nature—equilibrium (*sattva*), activity (*rajas*), and inertia (*tamas*) (*guṇas,* see commentary in aphorism I.16). These qualities do not always show themselves appropriately. For example, instead of being flooded with inertia when dropping off to sleep, we might experience overactivity, then, in the morning when this overactivity would be welcome, we are tired, and inertia predominates.

Once we recognize this, we can see it in others, though we may not always be able to alleviate this suffering. Discernment allows us to become aware of the mechanism and avoid its return, as the next aphorism tells us. In fact, everything can cause suffering for someone who lacks vigilance.

pariṇāmatāpasaṃskāraduḥkhairguṇavṛttivirodhācca duḥkhameva sarvaṃ vivekinaḥpariṇāma-tāpa-saṃskāra duḥkhaiḥ-guṇa-vṛtti-virodhāt-ca duḥkham-eva sarvaṃ vivekinaḥ

Pariṇāma: transformation, or change due to time, lapse of time, motivation. *Tāpa:* burn, grief, worry. *Saṃskāra:* impregnation of the mind, conditioning, habit. *Duḥkhaiḥ:* ache, pain, sadness. *Guṇa:* constituent qualities of nature, attributes. *Vṛtti:* activity, fluctuation, movement. *Virodhāt:* contradictory character, incompatibility, conflict, hostility. *Ca:* and. *Duḥkham:* suffering. *Eva:* assuredly, for sure. *Sarvam:* all. *Vivekinaḥ:* for the person of discernment, the sage.

Future suffering should be avoided.

Before acting, do I take time to ensure that it won't increase suffering?

Are my actions and commitments sufficiently well adjusted to keep me from making myself and others suffer?

Why do we dwell on past suffering, rather than trying to prevent future suffering?

Can we prevent future suffering (I.31)? When it occurs, what attitude should we have toward it?

As there is no life without joy and pain, how do we answer those who use this aphorism to avoid suffering by refusing to fully commit themselves in life?

Is it always better to hope for the best, while being prepared for the worst?

What is the connection between this aphorism and aphorism I.36?

This aphorism might seem a little simplistic. Who wants to suffer? However, it insists quite rightly that we can exercise prudence to prevent future suffering.

It emphasizes the warning given in the preceding aphorism. Awareness of what leads to suffering brings with it the will and the possibility to prevent it. Acting on existential suffering affects future suffering by working with the present mechanisms that later give rise to it (II.15). It means remaining vigilant about the motives behind today's actions, so they do not produce later suffering. That means three things:

- Do not aggravate suffering.
- Alleviate suffering, whenever possible.
- Prevent the return of suffering.

In this way, suffering can then present a positive aspect leading us to examine its causes and modify our behavior (II.3 and II.15). It becomes a factor of progression. This aphorism corresponds to a principal aim of yoga—to eliminate suffering.

heyaṃ duḥkhamanāgatam
heyaṃ duḥkham-anāgatam

Heyam: what (that which) is to be abandoned, avoided, rejected. *Duḥkham:* suffering, pain. *Anāgatam:* what has not yet happened or arrived.

The cause of pain is the union between the inner being who perceives and that which is perceived.

Can setbacks or the remarks of others help me to recognize lack of lucidity about myself?

How can I become impartial about myself?

How can a lack of impartiality lead to difficulty?

How does the union (saṃyoga), or confusion, presented here relate to ignorance (II.5) and the awareness of "I" (II.6)?

Does this aphorism imply that yoga, as a state of union, is above all a distinction between two levels of human nature?

Patañjali underlines the cause of suffering as confusion between two distinct levels of human nature, the spiritual principle (*draṣṭar*), and the material world (*dṛsyam,* II.6), the consequence of this confusion is lack of lucidity about oneself.

By definition, the spiritual principle is far removed from fluctuations, qualities, attributes, or time. The material universe, on the other hand, manifests itself at more or less subtle levels: the mineral, vegetable, and animal kingdoms; and the human race, including emotional, intellectual, and other levels.

The confusion between spiritual and material levels is even more pernicious when it becomes established in subtle, invisible domains, giving rise to mistaken impulses (*kleśas*). This aphorism implies that the lack of impartiality with regard to our deeper reality is at the root of all difficulties. That is why we must extricate ourselves from this mistaken union.

draṣṭṛdṛśyayoḥ saṃyogo heyahetuḥ
draṣṭṛ-dṛśyayoḥ saṃyogaḥ heya-hetuḥ

Draṣṭṛ: of the one who perceives or observes. *Dṛśyayoḥ:* of that which is perceived, the object. *Saṃyogaḥ:* union, reunion, close contact. *Heya:* that which is to be avoided, rejected. *Hetuḥ:* the cause.

II.18

What is perceived has clarity, movement, and inertia and is made up of the elements and the eleven senses. It can lead to sensory experience and to deliverance.

Does clarity, movement, or inertia predominate in my temperament?

How can I develop or diminish clarity, movement, or inertia when necessary?

What is the importance of the senses of perception and the senses of action in my relationship with the environment?

Do I hold the floor, or am I a listener?

Am I more inclined to plunge myself into sensory experience, or am I attracted by the absolute, the pure, or the afterlife?

Can awareness of this difference help me understand myself and others?

How can I live with the alternation between sensory experience and deliverance without inner conflict?

This aphorism and the next one make explicit one of the two entities that make up a human being—that which is perceived (*dṛśyam*). The *Sāṃkhya* system uses the term *prakṛti* (nature) for this entity. This entity is presented according to its characteristics, its components, and its double aim. Its characteristics take up once more the three constituent qualities of the nature of the *Sāṃkhya,* but in different terms (see the commentary in aphorism I.16).

ACCORDING TO YOGA	ACCORDING TO SĀṂKHYA
Prakāśa (clarity)	*Sattva* (purity)
Kriyā (movement)	*Rajas* (activity)
Sthiti (inertia)	*Tamas* (obscurity)

The components of matter are the five elements: ether, air, fire, water, and earth. According to the *Sāṃkhya-kārikā,* nature takes material form in these five basic elements. Each of the words that designate one of these elements must be taken in its widest sense:

- Ether (*akāśa*) is the notion of space, a void, and potential space.
- Air (*vāyu*) is the notion of gaseousness, of movement and displacement.
- Fire (*tejas*) is the notion of heat, temperature, transformation, and purification.
- Water (*āpas*) is the notion of liquid, fluidity, and flow.
- Earth (*pṛthivi*) is the notion of mass, solidity, and density.

These elements are perceived through:

- The three internal organs: thought (*buddhi*); the faculty of understanding (*ahaṃkāra*); and the faculty of coordination (*manas*). The last is also a sense organ.
- The ten sense organs, which include the five senses of perception—hearing, touch, sight, taste, smell—and the five senses of action—speech, grasping or holding, locomotion, excretion, and generation.

On the one hand, these organs permit enjoyment, sensory experience, and experimentation. On the other hand, we must go beyond them, to be free of them without rejecting them. This is the description, with no notion of relative values, of two types of relationship with reality. They may be connected in time, or by experimentation that leads to deliverance (as learning a language frees one from the school notebook and enables one to speak). The first relationship approaches suffering (*paritāpa*) and joy (*hlāda* II.14). The second, beatitude, or bliss (*ānanda* I.17), which transcends all duality between suffering and enjoyment.

prakāśakriyāsthitiśīlam bhūtendriyātmakaṃ
bhogapavargārthaṃ dṛśyam
prakāśa-kriyā- sthiti-śīlaṃ bhūta-indriya-ātmakaṃ
bhoga-apavarga-arthaṃ dṛśyam

Prakāśa: light, illumination, apparition. *Kriyā:* action, realization, activity. *Sthiti:* fixity, immobility, cessation. *Śīlam:* character, tendency. *Bhūta:* the five gross elements (ether, air, fire, water, earth). *Indriya:* the eleven sense organs including thought. *Ātmakam:* consisting in, composed of. *Bhoga:* enjoyment, experience. *Apavarga:* liberation, deliverance. *Artham:* the aim, function. *Dṛśyam:* that which is perceived, the object, the visible.

II.19

The origin and characteristics of things are perceived or not perceived.

Am I able to accept others' viewpoints as well as my own and see that they complement each other?

Is it easy for me to accept that my vision is limited?

How can the contents of this aphorism help me develop awareness or make choices?

Is this aphorism more likely to lead me to greater tolerance for the opinions of others or to a stronger affirmation of my own viewpoint?

How can I refine my perception in a concrete way?

This aphorism presents a notion that Chapter IV also addresses: the multiplicity of nature's manifestations. Their diversity implies two aspects: nature as a perceived object and the mind as an observing instrument, also integral to nature, that selects what it perceives from among innumerable possibilities.

In the relationship between the observer and the observed, we can make out two fields of observation. First, external peculiarities, at first glance (*viśeṣa*), either stand out clearly for the observer or escape notice. Secondly, the observer may or may not notice specific inner details linked to origin (*liṅga*). These differences come from the observer's mind rather than from the object under observation. They are related to the intrinsic quality of the observer—to his or her knowledge of the field being observed.

The teaching we can draw from this aphorism is that one never sees everything, that everyone perceives a given object differently, and that each new glimpse of the object is different, even though the observer remains the same.

viśeṣāviśeṣaliṅgamātrāliṅgāni guṇaparvāṇi
viśeṣa-aviśeṣa-liṅgamātra-aliṅgāni guṇa-parvāṇi

Viśeṣa: specific, particular, characteristic. *Aviśeṣa:* nonspecific, not particular, uncharacteristic. *Liṅgamātra:* differentiated. *Aliṅgāni:* undifferentiated. *Guṇa:* constituent qualities of nature, attributes. *Parvāṇi:* the stage, degree, division.

The perceiving entity can only perceive. It uses the mind to experiment, but remains unaltered itself.

Am I able to live each situation intensely, yet maintain cool appraisal?

Am I more suited to intensifying my engagement in an experience or keeping my distance?

Can this aphorism lead me to change the way I relate to others?

What is the difference between Īśvara (I.23) and the perceiving entity?

After focusing on the painful union between the two levels of human nature (II.17) and explaining that which is perceived (*dṛsyam*) in aphorisms II.18 and II.19, in this aphorism, Patañjali becomes more explicit about the perceiving entity (*draṣṭar*).

This spiritual principle, proper to every human being, is both related to matter and dissociated from it. This is like a mirror, which can reveal images without modifying its own nature. This spiritual entity uses the five mental activities—understanding, error, imagination, deep sleep, and memory—to exercise its perceiving faculty (I.6). The quality of perception, therefore, depends on the degree of clarity or dispersion in the mind.

Everything that impinges on the mind is a mental experience, whether conscious or unconscious, voluntary or involuntary—thoughts, feelings, sensations, and so on. For the perceiving entity to perceive and reveal itself in all its purity, we must control the mind. This is the aim of yoga (I.2).

draṣṭā dṛśimātraḥ śuddho 'pi pratyayānupaśyaḥ
draṣṭā dṛśimātraḥ śuddhaḥ-api pratyaya-anupaśyaḥ

Draṣṭā: entity who perceives, or observes. *Dṛśimātraḥ:* absolute vision, being nothing but vision. *Śuddhaḥ:* pure, clear, unmixed, irreproachable. *Api:* even, even though. *Pratyaya:* the experience made by the mind, idea, intellectual grasp, belief, faith. *Anupaśyaḥ:* perceived, continually observed.

II.21

What is perceived exists only to serve as object for the perceiving entity.

How can discovering that my life is not an end in itself, but a means of spiritual awakening, affect my personality, my relationships with others, and my objectives?

Can shifting my focus from the outcome of an action to the discovery of myself through action influence the result?

How can I avoid taking the means as an end?

Is it beneficial to ask myself what I have learned after every new experience?

The reality of the objective world, which comprises the body, mental faculties, thoughts, feelings, and the psyche as a whole, serves as a field of experience for the spiritual principle in each one of us. The objective world does not exist on its own account, but only to serve the inner being. The image of the bed, for example, does not exist in itself, but only to serve the one who sleeps in it (see also *Sāṃhya Kārikā 17, Gauḍapāda's* commentary). Without the inner being, the objective world would not show itself—it would not exist, having no reason in itself to be.

This is tantamount to saying that every circumstance in daily life is an experience in which consciousness, perception, or lucidity are more or less developed. If seeking perfection in an act is important, it is essential to continuously refine fundamental perception—the direct grasp of oneself and of others.

tadartha eva dṛśyasyātmā
tad-arthaḥ eva dṛśyasya-ātmā

Tad: this latter (designates draṣṭar: the perceiving entity in the preceding aphorism). *Arthaḥ:* aim, goal, object. *Eva:* assuredly, justly, precisely, correctly. *Dṛśyasya:* that which is perceived. *Ātmā:* proper nature, peculiar nature, essence.

What is perceived no longer exists for the perceiving entity once the intent is fulfilled, but it still exists to serve others.

What difficulty can arise if I become attached to an object that has fulfilled its mission (for example, learning the grammar that enabled me to speak a foreign language)?

What difficulty can arise if I never unite myself sufficiently with the perceived object (for example, neglect grammar)?

What do I understand about this opposition between the existence or nonexistence of perceived objects?

This aphorism further clarifies the preceding one. Since the function of any object is to serve a spiritual principle, it no longer has any reason to exist when it has fulfilled its function. It can, however, continue to exist through serving other beings. When a backward-bending yoga posture straightens someone's hunched back, it has then fulfilled its use to that person, but it can still help others or even the same person if the same problem later recurs.

If the manifested universe is a field of experience that allows us to develop our awareness, why should it still exist after it has reached its peak? Since communication depends on the sense organs, which belong to the manifested universe, the majority of beings still have need of it. Even if one goes beyond the preliminary stages of progress, it is necessary to keep them in mind in order to communicate with those still passing through them.

This high degree of liberation calls to mind the two categories of exceptional beings (*videha* and *prakṛtilayānam*) introduced in aphorism I.19 and the description of the liberated state in Chapter IV.

kṛtārthaṃ prati naṣṭamapyanaṣṭaṃ tadanyasādhāraṇatvāt
kṛta-arthaṃ prati naṣṭam-api-anaṣṭaṃ tad-anya-sādhāraṇatvāt

Kṛta: realized, accomplished. *Artham:* the aim. *Prati:* compared to, with regard to. *Naṣṭam:* disappeared, destroyed. *Api:* but, however. *Anaṣṭaṃ:* not destroyed. *Tad:* that (designated dṛśya: that which is perceived, in the preceding aphorism). *Anya:* other. *Sādhāraṇatvāt:* being in common.

II.23

The union of that which is perceived and the perceiving entity permits understanding of their respective faculties.

How can I begin to see that each experience, including my errors, can help me develop lucidity?

Can I overcome certain difficulties only by exploring or experiencing them, instead of running away from them?

When should I commit myself to an experience and when should I avoid getting involved?

How can I use even my lack of lucidity and cool appraisal as a means of evolution?

The potential for objective vision is always present in us. But, being too involved in ourselves, we clutter it with our subjective views. Our projections, emotions, and sentiments lead us astray.

This imperfect condition has a positive aspect. It pushes us to evolve with greater lucidity toward correct action and awareness of the two entities and their respective roles. This aphorism emphasizes that through our mistakes, we make progress. Aren't mistakes part of any apprenticeship?

Uniting with life in all its forms enables us to better grasp what life is about and who and what we are ourselves. In risking mistakes, we come to understand action and the way we behave in the course of action. This study of the *Yoga Sūtras* permits both understanding of the text and understanding of oneself.

svasvāmiśaktyoḥ svarūpopalabdhihetuḥ saṃyogaḥ
sva-svāmi-śaktyoḥ sva-rūpa-upalabdhi-hetuḥ saṃyogaḥ

Sva: that which is perceived, oneself. *Svāmi:* perceiving entity, master, owner. *Śaktyoḥ:* power, force, faculty. *Svarūpa:* proper, peculiar nature. *Upalabdhi:* acquisition, understanding. *Hetuḥ:* cause. *Saṃyogaḥ:* union, conjunction, reunion, close contact (between that which is perceived and the one who perceives).

The cause of this union is ignorance.

Do I grow in understanding every time I accept I am wrong?

Am I able to listen to others' opinions about me?

In a more general way, do I know how to use the mirror of others to find, improve, and enrich myself?

Does dissatisfaction motivate me to take such steps?

If we often lack objectivity, if we are too wrapped up in ourselves, the cause is ignorance (*avidyā*), introduced as the first cause of suffering in aphorism II.4 and defined in aphorism II.5.

This ignorance, or lack of lucidity about reality, is confusion, wherein we cling to distorted images. It is like the monkey that sees itself in a mirror and goes behind the mirror to find the other monkey it has just seen. We create such situations whenever we enclose ourselves in a mistaken opinion, or when having understood a reality, we forget it as soon as life no longer reminds us of it.

The cause of all our difficulties, then, is our stubbornly maintaining opinions that are not aligned with reality. Such an attitude, due to our lack of lucidity about ourselves and the world, becomes even more difficult to see when we are closely involved with people and things. One often sees more clearly in a professional relationship than in a personal one.

tasya heturavidyā
tasya hetuḥ-avidyā

Tasya: of this, about this (designates *saṃyoga:* union, quoted in the preceding aphorism). *Hetuḥ:* the cause, reason. *Avidyā:* ignorance.

II.25

When ignorance vanishes, so does union.
Its absence brings serenity.

Why must I let go of believing that I know everything in order to begin to know something?

What in me still stands in the way of this liberation?

What part do simplicity and humility play in opening up to this wisdom?

How will discovering this affect my health, my personality, and my relationships?

What is the difference between the contemplative state (Chapter I) and serenity?

This aphorism deals with ending ignorance and realizing serenity (*kaivalya,* title of Chapter IV). As ignorance gradually disappears, the perception of reality grows ever clearer. With clear-sightedness, the muddle of ideas ceases and beatitude—serenity—appears. Evoked here for the first time, serenity, the ultimate end of yoga, constitutes a state of happiness, peace, and everlasting compassion. Patañjali devotes the last chapter to this state.

tadabhāvātsaṃyogābhāvo hānaṃ taddṛśeḥ kaivalyam
tad-abhāvāt-saṃyoga-abhāvaḥ hānam tad-dṛśeḥ kaivalyam

Tad: this, this latter (designates the cause of ignorance (*avidyā,* II.24)). *Abhāvāt:* of the absence, of the disappearance. *Saṃyoga:* union, confusion, conjunction. *Abhāvaḥ:* absence, disappearance. *Hānam:* ceasing. *Tad:* of this, this latter (referring to *hānam:* ceasing). *Dṛśeḥ:* vision, clear-sightedness. *Kaivalyam:* serenity, beatitude, liberation.

Awareness of unequivocal discernment ends confused union.

Have improvements in my discernment, lucidity, and skill in active life enhanced my evolution?

If there is no apparent evolution, how should I change my outlook? Is discernment innate or acquired?

This aphorism and the preceding one describe a deep transformation. How will this affect my personal and professional conduct, my relationships with others, and my evolution?

Does this aphorism imply that I will not have any more setbacks and that I won't make any more mistakes, or does it imply that I will see them differently?

The previous aphorisms have studied ignorance as a cause of suffering. This particular aphorism presents a way of ending it by developing discernment, the faculty of discrimination, and seeing clearly what is essential, without ambiguity. Through this, one develops a lucid mind that perceives persons, situations, and problems objectively and positively.

Such discernment must be obvious and intervene in all options, ideas, and acts. It must also be permanent. It doesn't happen sporadically, it is constant. Such discrimination is fundamental to knowing and marking out one's evolution. It is a means of attaining the serenity evoked in the preceding aphorism.

vivekakhyātiraviplavā hānopāyaḥ
viveka-khyātiḥ-aviplavā hāna-upāyaḥ

Viveka: discernment, discrimination, distinction (between). *Khyātiḥ:* apprehension, recognition. *Aviplavā:* absence of confusion, total clarity. *Hāna:* ending, ceasing (implicitness of *saṃyoga:* union). *Upāyaḥ:* the means, method, way.

II.27

The ultimate wisdom that emerges has seven stages.

Am I ready to acknowledge that I have a problem?

Am I ready to ask for help? If not, what prevents me from taking these first steps?

On my own, can I:

- *discover the causes of my problems?*
- *determine a goal that will help get me clear of them?*
- *choose means to attain my goal that suits my personality?*

In handing down yoga, is it useful or harmful to inform the student:

- *of his or her problems and their causes?*
- *of the goal of yoga?*
- *only of the means to free oneself?*

What care must I take in applying the first four stages of wisdom to the subtle or hidden level of reality?

Do the seven stages of wisdom apply to other fields—teaching, for example?

What is the relationship between this ultimate wisdom and that presented in aphorism I.48?

What is the relationship between this aphorism and the recommendation made concerning suffering in II.16?

The sevenfold wisdom emerges as a direct result of discernment. According to T.K.V. Desikachar, the seven stages of the way of wisdom are:

1. Becoming aware of suffering (*duḥkha*)
2. Recognizing and removing causes of suffering (*hetu*)
3. Determining a goal
4. Having clear vision of the means
5. Applying these first four stages as a whole to a manifested level—the general exterior and physical level
6. Applying these same four stages as a whole to an unmanifested level—the interior, subtle, psychological, or spiritual level
7. Becoming aware of the spiritual principle that allows the whole process—complete liberation.

The first four items are steps, taken chronologically. The last three steps encompass the different levels, from the grossest to the more subtle.

1. Accept that suffering is real and that it comes from yourself. This is preliminary to all evolution, whether you accept your daily mistakes, personal problems, or metaphysically recognize your own suffering (II.16 and II.17). No one else can take these steps for you. Even when the causes of suffering are external—coming from nature or from others—very often they are also in you.
2. Recognize that words, actions, or behavior can cause suffering. Then dig deeper to discover the root of the cause in one of the five categories of erroneous impulses set out in aphorism II.3.
3. Determine a clear objective that provides you with positive anchorage to help you avoid aggravating the suffering that comes from recognizing causes.
4. Clarify your vision of the means. Several means can lead to positive transformation, but choosing the one that best serves your transformation requires discernment (II.26).
5. After working through these four stages on the physical level with a guide (working on a health problem, for example), as you gradually evolve toward autonomy, you can begin to follow these four stages of wisdom on your own to address other physical or general difficulties.
6. Then, it becomes possible to approach the deeper, subtler sphere of your psychology with regard to the Absolute—first with a guide, then later with some autonomy.
7. The last stage of wisdom is a growing awareness of the perceiving entity, who allowed the steps we took toward serenity.

tasya saptadhā prāntabhūmiḥ prajñā
tasya saptadhā prānta-bhūmiḥ prajñā

Tasya: of this latter (designates *hanopayaḥ*: the way that leads to cessation, quoted in the preceding aphorism). *Saptadha:* seven stages, sevenfold. *Prāntabhūmiḥ:* ultimate, final. *Prajña:* wisdom, deep knowledge, inner knowledge.

Eliminating impurity through continued practice of the eight limbs of yoga brings discernment and clear perception.

Am I ready to undertake the yoga of the eight limbs:

- *with a guide?*
- *as a daily, continuous practice?*
- *with steadfastness?*

Have the steps I've taken in yoga brought me:

- *better day-to-day discernment?*
- *clearer thought?*
- *fewer negative impulses (kleṣas)?*
- *improved suppleness?*

What is the difference between discrimination that stems from regular practice, including the eight limbs of yoga, and that which certain people instinctively possess?

Practicing the eight limbs of yoga (set out in the following aphorism) establishes discernment. Such evolution calls for a guide and for gradual, continual progress in a daily practice that aims for steadfastness. The impurities—the five types of disturbance set out in aphorism II.3—are gradually reduced to a latent state. It is then that well-founded discernment appears, the aptitude of spontaneously choosing the best option in all circumstances. Thought is clear, thus, the rupture between the spiritual and material aspects that make up our nature (II.26) becomes clear.

yogāṅgānuṣṭhānādaśuddhikṣaye jñānadīptirāvivekakhyāteḥ
yoga-aṅga-anuṣṭhānāt-aśuddhi-kṣaye jñāna-dīptiḥ-ā-viveka-khyateḥ

Yoga: of yoga. *Aṅga:* the limbs, part. *Anuṣṭhānāt:* by the execution, action in conformity with, religious practice. *Aśuddhi:* impurity. *Kṣaye:* in destruction, diminishing, end. *Jñāna:* wisdom, deep knowledge. *Dīptiḥ:* light, radiance. *Ā:* up to. *Viveka:* discernment. *Khyāteḥ:* in apprehending, in recognizing.

The eight limbs of yoga are: respect toward others, self-restraint, posture, breath control, detaching at will from the senses, concentration, meditation, and contemplation.

Do I prefer certain limbs of yoga to others?

Do I tend to forget, reject, or fear certain limbs?

Is my attitude to the eight limbs evolving?

Can I focus only on one limb to the exclusion of the others?

Which of the eight limbs of yoga can be taught, orally or otherwise?

How do the eight limbs relate to each other?

Patañjali lists eight limbs of yoga, thus excluding any others. The order of listing reflects the different levels of human being, from our relationship with the outer world to the most subtle aspects of ourselves, from the outside to the inside.

- The first limb concerns difficulties in relationships with others.
- The second limb proposes guidelines for personal daily behavior.
- The third limb intervenes on the physical level—the body—through posture practice.
- The fourth limb helps us better manage the energies that animate the body, linked to the emotions by the practice of breath control.
- The fifth limb allows us to regain control of the senses to prevent them from dragging us in their wake.
- The last three limbs concern consciousness and describe three progressive stages on the way to inner peace or spiritual liberation.

The listing of the eight limbs does not correspond to a necessary chronological order of steps one must follow in yoga, since different personalities will prefer a different order. However, the steps in yoga often follow the order below:

1. Posture practice and breath control can become a practice in themselves and improve relations not only with oneself, but with others as well.

2. As concentration grows, along with posture practice and breath control, one develops the ability to control sensory perceptions, actions, and thoughts.
3. The last two limbs follow successively, dependng on the preceding results.

The end of Chapter II and the beginning of Chapter III present the eight limbs.

yamaniyamāsanaprāṇāyāmapratyāhāradhāraṇādhyāna - samādhayo 'ṣṭāvaṅgani
yama-niyama-āsana-prāṇāyāma-pratyāhāra-dhāraṇā-dhyāna-samādhayaḥ-aṣṭau-aṅgāni

Yama: attitudes toward the surroundings and toward others. *Niyama:* attitudes toward oneself. *Āsana:* practice of physical exercises, of postures. *Prāṇāyāma:* practice of breathing exercises, breath control. *Pratyāhāra*: the withdrawal of the senses from objects, mastery of the senses. *Dhāraṇā:* concentration, aptitude for directing the mental function. *Dhyāna:* meditation, aptitude of developing, without fail, interactions with what we are trying to understand. *Samādhayaḥ:* contemplation, complete integration with the object of understanding. *Aṣṭau:* eight. Aṅgāni: limbs, parts.

The principles of respect for others include nonviolence, truth, honesty, moderation, and noncovetousness.

Which of these five principles do I find easy to follow, and which are more difficult?

Is it ever desirable to focus on just one of these principles to the exclusion of the others?

For me, are these principles a practice, mental vigilance, or progressive discovery?

Can we see in these principles a chain of causes and effects from the first to the last?

How can I avoid moralizing in my understanding and presentation of these precepts?

These principles concern relationships with others, but do not exclude the relationship with the self.

- Respect for all beings and all things must permeate all levels. It can never include physical violence (wounds and blows), verbal aggression (shouts, perfidious language, and slander), or behavior that leads to ill effects (intolerance or the desire to shock), especially toward the weak. It begins with respect for one's own body, including not impairing one's health by abnormal practice of postures or breath control.
- Respect for truth encompasses all modes of communication, words, gestures, writings, and so on. The *Mahābhārata* defines this attitude thus: "Truth should be told when agreeable, should be said agreeably, and truth should not be said that does harm; however, never lie to give pleasure."
- Respect for what belongs to others, or honesty and probity, consists in not unduly taking for oneself goods of any nature whatsoever—material, intellectual, or any other kind. For example, do not adopt someone else's ideas without crediting him or her, nor acquire something without compensation and the agreement of the one who concedes it.
- Respect for moderation is necessary on the profane and the religious levels. It is the correct balancing of actions, desires, thoughts, and feelings, and channeling them first toward the quest for the absolute or higher realization.
- Respect for a well-founded desire, or noncovetousness, consists in not seeking to possess undue or superfluous goods. This includes not accumulating ill-considered and useless gifts, gratifications, or perquisites.

Sometimes situations arise in which one might have to choose one principle of respect over another. For example, a person with terminal cancer who is in a weak psychological state might ask for the truth about his or her chances of survival and the number of weeks left to live. Should the principle of nonviolence be respected by giving no reply, so as not to aggravate distress, or should the truth be respected?

The principles are listed in the order of priority. The first principle, nonviolence, encompasses all the others. It has priority over the second, the second over the third, and so on. In other words, respect nonviolence before veracity, and veracity before honesty, moderation, and noncovetousness. This hierarchy is well demonstrated in the axiom from the Mahābhārata: It is better to tell the sick person what he or she can bear with gentleness, and as agreeably as possible.

ahiṃsāsatyāsteyabrahmacaryāparigrahā yamāḥ
ahiṃsā-satya-asteya-brahmacarya-aparigrahāḥ yamāḥ

Ahiṃsā: nonviolence, abstaining from harm, respect for life. *Satya:* veracity, truth, authenticity, reality. *Asteya:* not stealing. *Brahmacarya:* moderation, continence, quest for truth. *Aparigrahāḥ:* noncovetousness, lack of greed for wealth, lack of greed. *Yamāḥ:* chiefly, attitudes toward the surroundings (secondarily, attitudes toward oneself).

When unaffected by social or geographic considerations, or considerations of time or circumstances, these principles are universal. They are the supreme ideals.

What factors influence my respect for these principles: society, geography, the times I live in, or specific circumstances?

Regardless of the particular form it takes, does the teaching of yoga always imply absolute respect for these principles?

The ideal realization of these principles of respect has universal value. In daily life, however, external or internal restraints can limit their realization. Often they are modulated by where one lives and the climate, the time in which one lives, and finally, social, family, or personal circumstances. For example, respecting nonviolence is different for a priest and a soldier in time of war.

For those who have not mastered their instinctive or emotional reactions, these principles remain something to be attained little by little. For those who have mastered themselves, these principles induce a contemplation and union with God—we can say they become religious vows (*vratam*).

This aphorism presents a universal ethic that is very close to the Judeo-Christian one. Through what is unsaid, it leaves a place for accepting specific moral codes, which are stages in the life of the individual.

Moral codes and ethics here imply respect for certain principles that favor the inner evolution of the individual, and not conventional respect for a given religious or social rite.

jātideśakālasamayānavacchinnāḥ sārvabhaumā
mahāvratam
jāti-deśa-kāla-samaya-anavacchinnāḥ sārva-bhaumāḥ
mahā-vratam

Jāti: birth, rank, caste. *Deśa:* place, region. *Kāla:* time, destiny. *Samaya:* circumstances. *Anavacchinnāḥ:* not limited by. *Sārvabhaumāḥ:* in all the earth, everywhere. *Mahā:* great. *Vratam:* the rule, observance, vow.

II.32

The five personal principles of positive action are purity, contentment, a disciplined life, study of the sacred texts, and worship of God.

Which of these five principles do I find easy to respect, and which are difficult to attain?

How can I learn to respect these principles and others without sinking into moralizing and disciplinary attitudes?

Can a strong focus on one of these principles conflict with the others, or even the principles of respect listed in aphorism II.30?

Is there a necessary chronological order to the five personal principles of positive action?

Are the last three principles—discipline, study, and worship of God—part of daily practice, even though they seem more related to the yoga of action (II.1)?

Purity, physical as well as mental, is our first duty to the body and to the mind. It comprises external and internal physical cleanliness, that is to say, detoxification practices, as well as intellectual and moral rectitude.

Contentment is a positive attitude, reasoned or not, toward past, present, and future events. It is more than just passive satisfaction. It aims at balancing the psyche. We can best measure our aptitude for respecting this principle when circumstances are unfavorable.

The last three principles—a disciplined life, study of the sacred texts, and worship of God—again take up the three elements of the yoga of action presented in aphorism II.1. Here, they have a slightly different meaning: They are intrinsic to our daily, personal discipline:

- A disciplined life that aims for mental and physical balance is the practice of moderation in everything: sleep, work, rest, leisure, food, and human relationships.
- Daily study of the sacred texts includes reciting, intoning, or chanting them. It requires progressive apprenticeship. With no preconceptions, it aims at progressive discovery of oneself.
- Worship is an attitude of accepting what transcends us—allowing access to a higher force. A nonbeliever can open him- or herself to this surprising energy by observing the mystery of life and admiring and respecting those who have achieved exceptional great works during their lives.

These five principles are not independent of each other. Purity is the most important and produces the others. It leads to contentment, which favors respect for a disciplined life. This framework supports study of the sacred texts and facilitates worship of a higher force.

śaucasaṃtoṣatapaḥsvādhyāyeśvarapraṇidhānāni niyamāḥ
śauca-saṃtoṣa-tapaḥ-svādhyāya-īśvara-praṇidhānāni niyamāḥ

Śauca: purity, purification, cleanliness. *Saṃtoṣa:* contentment. *Tapaḥ:* ascesis (discipline), austere practice, ardor, fervor. *Svādhyāya:* reading or chanting sacred texts. *Īśvara-praṇidhānāni:* devotion to the Lord, positive behavior and the ritual act of devotion. *Niyamāḥ:* observing positive actions with regard to self.

II.33

When harassed by doubt, cultivate the opposite mental attitude.

Do I take time to think things over before acting, especially when I am not sure which direction to take?

Could I use this means, even if only after the event, to understand the reason for certain setbacks?

What qualities must I foster to favor this line of action?

After addressing the principles of respect for oneself and others (II.30 to II.32), Patañjali devotes two aphorisms to presenting a way of practicing them.

Disrespect for these principles leads to inner conflicts, particularly when we hesitate over priorities. Is it better, for example, to speak the whole truth, or to remain nonviolent?

This method does not lead us to suppress contradictory impulses, but to work back to their source, so we can understand them better, analyze them, foresee their negative effects, and start again on a healthier basis. Don't they say to think twice about what we say before we speak?

It is a way of looking for a less emotional, less intellectual grasp of reality—a grasp that is deeper, more intuitive, and in the end, more judicious and correct (*vicāra*).

vitarkabādhane pratipakṣabhāvanam
vitarka-bādhane pratipakṣa-bhāvanam

Vitarka: doubt, discussion, supposition, movement of thought. *Bādhane:* oppression, harassment, torment. *Pratipakṣa:* opposite side, opposing part. *Bhāvanam:* state of mind.

Cultivating the opposite mental attitude is realizing that it is our own impatience, greed, anger, or aberration that leads us to think, provoke, and approve conflicting thoughts, such as violence. The intensity of such thoughts may be weak, medium, or strong, but their consequences, ever self-perpetuating, are always suffering and ignorance.

Is this mode of analysis best used when the problem first appears, or later, when the problem has either intensified or abated?

Am I equally responsible if I act directly, if I delegate, or if I simply approve or let something ride?

Do my difficulties come from impatience, greed, haste, or anger? Or do they come from drowsiness, aberration, or inattentiveness?

Is it easy to link these conflicts with painful problems?

Is it possible that two or three causes of conflicting thoughts can come into play simultaneously?

What does it mean to say that negative consequences last forever?

What is the connection between this aphorism and aphorism II.10?

In this aphorism, Patañjali tells us how to escape contradictions among the five principles. He proposes analyzing the origin, cause, strength, and negative results of confusion. These different elements can combine in numerous ways that correspond to the sources of suffering (II.3).

This excellent method enables us to reverse the causes of suffering by accepting the negative value of our attitude; appreciating its gravity; searching for the feeling at its origin; determining our own share of responsibility; and, lastly, meditating on the never-ending dimension of negative effects.

As far as the causes are concerned, consuming eagerness and greed (*lobha*) include all greed, impatience, and haste in reflection and action. Anger (*krodha*) corresponds to any attitude, thought, or words that arouse one to passion. Aberration (*moha*) is the lack of reflection due to inertia, drowsiness, dreaminess, and illusion.

Turning the mental attitude in the other direction does not merely replace a feeling with its opposite (for example, replacing violence with nonviolence). Rather, it has us swim against the current to go back to its source and accept the evidence of its negative, perpetual effects. It then becomes possible to envisage another attitude or option while there is still time, so we can be positive, efficient, and peaceful.

vitarkā hiṃsādayaḥ kṛtakāritānumoditālobhakrodhamohapūrvakā mṛdumadhyādhimātrā duḥkhājñānānantaphalā iti pratipakṣabhāvanam

vitarkāḥ hiṃsā-ādayaḥ kṛta-kārita-anumoditāḥ lobha-krodha-moha-pūrvakāḥ mṛdu-madhya-adhimātrāḥ duḥkha-ajñāna-ananta-phalāḥ iti pratipakṣa-bhāvanam

Vitarkāḥ: doubts, contrary movements of thought. *Hiṃsā:* harming, creating damage, doing evil. *Ādayaḥ:* etcetera. *Kṛta:* done, accomplished (by oneself). *Kārita:* caused, occasioned, provoked. *Anumoditāḥ:* approved, authorized, let be. *Lobha:* consuming eagerness; greed, especially for wealth; haste. *Krodha:* anger, fury. *Moha:* aberration, loss of consciousness, hallucination, illusion. *Pūrvakāḥ:* provoked by, due to. *Mṛdu:* slight (degree). *Madhya:* medium (degree). *Adhimātrāḥ:* strong (degree), intense. *Duḥkha:* pain, suffering, affliction. *Ajñāna:* lack of knowledge, ignorance. *Ananta:* the infinite, eternal. *Phalāḥ:* the fruit of, result. *Iti:* here, end. *Pratipakṣa:* opposite side, contrary part. *Bhāvanam:* state of mind, mental attitude.

Around one who is solidly established in nonviolence, hostility disappears.

Am I more of an aggressive person or a victim of others?

How can I soften my temperament without repressing my aggression?

Do I tend to mask my weaknesses or timidity with nonviolence?

How do I respect both nonviolence and an ascetic life in a setting that is opposed to them?

Why is nonviolence the first and most important of the principles to respect with regard to others?

How does this respect for life engender the principles that follow it?

Patañjali devotes eleven aphorisms (II.35 to II.45) to defining principles with regard to others (*yamas*) and to oneself (*niyamas*). He does it skillfully, presenting them by their positive effects. These objectives can throw light on evolving toward the attitude concerned.

The first precept, respect for all beings and all things, calms aggressive impulses in those who, mentally or physically, are in contact with someone who has eliminated violence from his or her thoughts.

Violence toward another is not merely physical, but shows itself in actions, speech, dress, and thoughts. Being truly established in nonviolence involves all these elements.

The nonviolence that then blossoms should not be confused with cowardice or abandoning one's responsibilities. Neither should it be used to dominate or manipulate others. Quite the contrary, it places one at the service of others and helps one assume responsibilities.

ahiṃsāpratiṣṭhāyāṃ tatsaṃnidhau vairatyāgaḥ
ahiṃsā-pratiṣṭhāyāṃ tat-saṃnidhau vaira-tyāgaḥ

Ahiṃsā: nonviolence, abstaining from evil, respect for life. *Pratiṣṭhāyāṃ:* solid establishment, stability, foundation. *Tat:* this latter (the yogi who respects the principle of nonviolence). *Saṃnidhau:* in the neighborhood, near, presence. *Vaira:* animosity, hostility, discord, hate. *Tyāgaḥ:* abandonment, disappearance, leaving.

II.36

For one established in truth, the result fits the action.

Do I often blurt out the truth even if it is painful, or hide the truth through self-interest, fear, or weakness?

How can I avoid:

- *making promises that I can't keep?*
- *speaking a truth that has a negative result?*

Can I settle myself firmly in truth immediately, or must I slowly readjust with regard to family, profession, and so on?

Does this aphorism induce one to be more or less talkative?

Can words, gestures, and attitudes oppose each other? What is the result of action in that case?

Does expressing the truth always reinforce confidence?

Does veracity (satyam) imply correct perception (ṛtam, I.48)?

Veracity covers several domains: what we express, what we don't express, and how we express.

Veracity presupposes nonviolence and "if the truth is to be told, take care to tell it agreeably, and not tell it when it is negative, though one should never lie simply to give pleasure" (see II.30).

According to this aphorism, the acts of someone who really respects the truth will be powerfully and perfectly effective: What is said will be realized, what is done will be exemplary. There is correlation between the word, the action, and its result.

In several traditions, truth is with God—in the Gospel, "I am the Way, the Truth, the Life"—in *Chāndogya Upaniṣad,* truth is Being, that is, God. Truth is a fundamental concept. Respecting it is an exacting discipline that requires perfect fidelity and coherence among intention, speech, the action, and its results.

satyapratiṣṭhāyāṃ kriyāphalāśrayatvam
satya-pratiṣṭhāyāṃ kriyā-phala-āśrayatvam

Satya: veracity, truth, authenticity. *Pratiṣṭhāyām:* solid establishment, foundation. *Kriyā:* action, realization. *Phala:* effect, result. *Āśrayatvam:* that a close relationship exists.

All the jewels appear for one who is firmly set in honesty.

Is my honesty material, intellectual, or spiritual?

Do others trust me easily?

Are there different kinds of respect for honesty, depending on the type of relationship: family, friendly, social, professional, or others?

How can I speak and write in a way that honors my work—my own ideas—as my own, yet still honors the sources and inspiration behind my expression?

How can I test the honesty of my relationship with God?

A mystic once said, "Every rich man is dishonest, or the son of a dishonest man." How are we to understand that?

Not stealing means not taking or receiving anything without agreement or giving something in exchange. The expression "all the jewels" means the best of everything in every sphere: material, intellectual, or spiritual. On the simplest level, honesty and uprightness attract confidence in all emotional and professional relations, and so on.

Even though establishing oneself in honesty and uprightness gives access to all the jewels, accepting or possessing them is not always desirable. Noncovetousness (II.30) implies this. It is the same with indiscretions about one's possessions, where the ego often rears its head (II.6).

While being honest in the sphere of material goods may not be too difficult, determining and honoring great intellectual and spiritual probity is a more delicate affair. Using friends' notes, forgetting to include a bibliography, or assuming a status that doesn't tally with one's inner evolution, are just a few of the traps.

steyapratiṣṭhāyāṃ sarvaratnopasthānam
asteya-pratiṣṭhāyāṃ sarva-ratna-upasthānam

Asteya: not stealing. *Pratiṣṭhāyām:* solid establishment, foundation. *Sarva:* all, of all kinds. *Ratna:* jewel, pearl, precious stone or object. *Upasthānam:* approaching.

II.38

Vitality appears in one who is firmly set in moderation.

Am I in good shape or am I tired or tense?

Do I tend to relax, get bottled up, or waste my energy?

Must I experience expansiveness or intensity in emotional, sensual, or sexual relationships before I can live in moderation? Is this also the case with my partner(s)?

Can one person in a couple live in moderation without his or her partner agreeing to it or sharing it?

Is moderation valid if it appears only in certain spheres, for example in the sensual, but not in the emotional?

Does age play an important part in this concept?

Can a believer be immoderate in his or her dealings with God?

Moderation creates a harmonious relationship among the different forms of energy that animate the body: emotional, sensual, sexual, physical, and the more subtle energy of thought.

The Sanskrit word translated as "moderation" (*brahmacarya*) designates amongst other things, adolescence, the period of life allotted to study. It means making one's way toward God. This indicates that chastity, whether monastic or conjugal, can be the source of high spiritual felicity.

Such moderation in use of one's energy—leaving physical pleasure and psychological well-being behind—can only make it stronger. Good management of it often passes progressively from quantity to quality and from egoism to altruism.

The Sanskrit word translated as "vital force" (*vīrya*) also means sperm. Continence is a way of resolving sterility.

brahmacaryapratiṣṭhāyāṃ vīryalābhaḥ
brahmacarya-pratiṣṭhāyāṃ vīrya-lābhaḥ

Brahmacarya: moderation, continence, search for truth. *Pratiṣṭhāyām:* solid establishment, stability, foundation. *Vīrya:* vitality, valiance, vigor, energy *Lābhaḥ:* finding, obtaining, gain.

One who perseveres on the path of noncovetousness gains deep understanding of the meaning of life.

Are my possessions adequate for my needs?

Do I tend to accumulate things or desire material goods, knowledge, or useless holy objects?

How can I prevent the upkeep, protection, and renewal of my possessions from overwhelming me?

Should a minimum of ownership precede noncovetousness?

Does noncovetousness imply a life of poverty?

How can I tell whether the absence of wordly goods is a sign of noncovetousness or of repressed covetousness?

What is the relationship between noncovetousness, attachment (II.7), and nonattachment (I.15 and I.16)?

Noncovetousness consists in not acquiring superfluous goods nor desiring them, nor accepting gifts beyond reasonable limits. The notion of superfluous goods varies with the individual and his or her social and family position.

The more one owns, the more one needs to protect it. Accepting more than is necessary and acquiring more and more goods, knowledge, relationships, and mystical states, clutters the mind and keeps it from grasping the source of things and the motivations and reasons for our life.

When the mind no longer worries about acquiring and keeping goods, we understand where we come from, where we are, and where we are going. We discover the meaning of existence, which can bring us:

- liberty that proceeds from a thorough appraisal of our situation and its origin, of our conditioning, and of our possible choices
- a moral force that issues from knowledge of our destiny

aparigrahasthairye janmakathaṃtā saṃbodhaḥ
aparigraha-sthairye janma-kathaṃtā saṃbodhaḥ

Aparigraha: Lack of covetousness, impatience, and greed. *Sthairye:* firmness, constancy, perseverance, perfection in. *Janma:* birth, origin, existence. *Kathaṃtā:* the how and why. *Saṃbodhaḥ:* total knowledge, deep understanding.

II.40

Purity protects one's body and brings nonphysical relationships with others.

How much time should I spend each day washing, dressing, and practicing my yoga or any other discipline that aims at getting rid of impurities (tapas, II.1)?

Should I change the amount of time I spend on any of these?

How can I prevent self-care from turning into egocentrism—or contemplation of my navel?

Can excessive cleanliness turn against me?

How is this aphorism related to the confusion of the pure and the impure (avidyā, II.5)?

This aphorism introduces the first and most important of the personal principles of positive action: purity. It presents awareness at the level of the body, whether your own or another's. The mental aspect is the object of the next aphorism.

Physical purity goes beyond simply cleansing the body, or cleansing impurities through posture practice and breathing exercises (*tapaḥ,* II.1). It allows us to evaluate the need for constant, repetitive care of the physical and brings out the ephemeral character of the body, diminishing our attachment to it. It is understood that there is an essential inner dimension beyond physical appearance. Real communication with others is then situated at this inner level.

Purity allows us to develop and maintain good health. If this is excessive, however, and becomes an end in itself, it can be destructive. It could lead to refusing contact with others, creating obstacles to human relations and compassion, whereas, when well understood, it favors them.

śaucātsvāṅgajugupsāparairasaṃsargaḥ
śaucāt-svāṅga-jugupsā-paraiḥ-asaṃsargaḥ

Śaucāt: purity, purification, cleanliness. *Sva:* his, her, proper, own. *Aṅga:* the body. *Jugupsā:* care, keeping, protecting. *Paraiḥ:* others. *Asaṃsargaḥ:* unmixed, not mixing.

Then, purity, clarity, and well-being of the spirit come to flower, as well as concentration, mastery of the eleven sense organs, and perception of the inner being.

Can I estimate the purity of my feelings and my thoughts by listening to the remarks of others or taking advice? Or should I take time to observe and analyze myself?

Can I enhance this purity by reducing inertia and drowsiness (tamas) or cutting down overactivity (rajas)?

Is yoga an eliminatory process for me?

How does purity of the mind, as described here, relate to veracity (II.36), well-being, and contentment (II.42)?

This aphorism leaves the bodily aspect (II.40) behind and addresses purity on the mental and spiritual levels. Purity is, therefore, both physical and mental. The first effects are shown in the development of understanding, clarity, and balance (*sattva* I.16) as opposed to inertia (*tamas*), or agitation (*rajas*). The *sattva* state of mind is accompanied by well-being and peace.

There is no temptation to flit from one thing to another. This is concentration and control of sensory perceptions and actions—the vision of the very essence of Being. The vision is clear in any situation. Purity, physical as well as mental, is an important aspect of evolution toward true self-realization.

sattvaśuddhisaumanasyaikāgryendriyajayātmadarśana-yogyatvāni ca

sattva-śuddhi-saumanasya-ekāgrya-indriyajaya-ātma-darśana-yogy-atvāni ca

Sattva: the mind at peace, equilibrium, balance. *Śuddhi:* purification; purity. *Saumanasya:* sentiment of well-being, good humor. *Ekāgrya:* focusing. *Indriya:* the eleven sense organs. *Jaya:* victory, mastery. *Ātma:* inner being, essence. *Darśana:* vision, understanding. *Yogyatvāni:* aptitude for. *Ca:* and.

II.42

Contentment brings supreme happiness.

Am I always happy and smiling, whatever happens?

Can self-satisfaction hide cowardice or a refusal to assume responsibilities (why change if one is happy)?

Can I become content through:

- *seeing my own actions and those of others in a positive light?*
- *always seeking a reason to be happy?*

How does contentment relate to or affect the dominating factors of ego (asmita) or fear (abhiniveśa)?

Can contentment bring success, or is commitment to success immaterial?

What is the relationship between contentment and smiling?

How does contentment relate to serenity (I.17), calmness (I.37), and noncovetousness (II.39)?

Contentment comes from mental well-being (*saumanasya*) that moves us to consider the positive in all beings and situations. Often, our frustrations come from regrets, agitation, suffering, or comparing ourselves with others. Focusing on what others have—or don't have, for that matter—instead of nourishing gratitude, leads to everlasting discontent.

Contentment is a dynamic and constructive attitude that brings us to look at things in a new way. It calms the mind, bringing a flowering of subtle joy and inner serenity that are independent of all outside influences and perishable things. It is essential for self-confidence, for succeeding in our personal endeavors, and for relationships, education, teaching, and therapy.

It is very difficult, however, to sustain contentment. Though it may be easier to be happy when we are successful, only an exceptional soul remains positive in the midst of adverse currents. Contentment means looking at every event with a smile. It helps to have a good sense of humor.

saṃtoṣādanuttamaḥ sukhalābhaḥ
saṃtoṣāt-anuttamaḥ sukha-lābhaḥ

Saṃtoṣāt: through or by contentment. *Anuttamaḥ:* the strongest. *Sukha:* of happiness, joy. *Lābhaḥ:* obtaining, gain.

By eliminating impurity, a disciplined life brings perfection and mastery to the body and the eleven sense organs.

Is my daily life well-balanced on all levels—do I get enough time for thought, leisure, eating, exercise, sleep, yoga, and other practices? If not, how can I find a happy medium?

Does reducing impurity help me to progress? What conclusion can I draw?

What is the relationship between contentment, which implies acceptance, and discipline, which aims at eliminating impurity?

Can I achieve this discipline only through will?

Can overzealous discipline interfere with eliminating impurity?

Does this aphorism encourage reevaluation of my practice of discipline, if after several years, I still have not realized physical plenitude or begun to master the senses?

How can I prevent perfection and mastery of the body and the sense organs from becoming an end in itself?

In this case, a disciplined life is a well-balanced ascetic medium that satisfies the real needs of being by taking care of body and mind without encumbering them with harmful or useless elements.

It means doing away with anything that hinders the functioning of the body and the eleven sense organs (see II.18). We attain this by keeping a good balance, first physically, then mentally, by being disciplined about food, sleep, exercise, work, and time for thought. We manage both the quantity and quality of our energy.

Healthy body and mind efficiently fulfill their roles as tools and prepare the way for consciousness in its plenitude, and the awakening of the heart.

kāyendriyasiddhiraśuddhikṣayāttapasaḥ
kāya-indriya-siddhiḥ-aśuddhi-kṣayāt-tapasaḥ

Kāya: the body. *Indriya:* the eleven sense organs, including thought. *Siddhiḥ:* power, perfection. *Aśuddhi:* impurity. *Kṣayāt:* by the destruction, elimination. *Tapasaḥ:* discipline, asceticism, austerity.

II.44

Union with the chosen divinity comes from the study of self through the sacred texts.

Do I devote time each day to reciting, studying, and meditating on an inspired text?

Can I do this without guidance in the beginning?

How do I choose a guide?

Do I become conscious of my limitations as I draw nearer to God, or do I draw nearer to God when I become conscious of my limitations?

Can certain kinds of self-reflection be premature?

Can we ever overdo self-reflection?

The Yoga Sūtras were written in a time and culture that emphasized the sacred. Contemporary Western culture is secular and sacredness that does not conform to accepted religion is often rejected. In such a context, what word can replace "divinity" (devata) in this aphorism?

The Sanskrit word translated as "study of self through the sacred texts" (*svādhyāya*) represents the recitation of the texts handed down by tradition. These texts are recognized as bearers of wisdom because they are revealed by God, and self-reflection using these texts is a starting point.

Such reflection implies questioning oneself over a long period. Sacred texts enable us to better understand the self and to discover our limitations, revealing the hidden side of things—the subtle universe of causes.

In this way, the recitation and assiduous study of the *Yoga Sūtras,* and any sacred text, allows a finer view of life and of self—it allows union with knowledge. A similar idea is expressed in aphorism I.39.

svādhyāyādiṣṭadevatāsaṃprayogaḥ
svādhyāyāt-iṣṭa-devatā-saṃprayogaḥ

Svādhyāyāt: through reading and chanting sacred texts. *Iṣṭa:* desired, chosen. *Devatā:* divinity. *Saṃprayogaḥ:* union, fusion.

Contemplation and its powers are attained through worship of God.

What is the role of faith in my life?

Even if I do not believe in God, have I looked up to anyone (my mother and father, a teacher, a wise person, a philosopher, or a writer)?

How can it help me to believe that there is always someone superior to me?

Why does confidence in a superior being lead to receiving greater powers from that being?

How can I prevent my devotion from turning into superstition or harmful zeal?

Is emotion important for my own concept of the absolute?

Is this aphorism useful for an agnostic or an atheist?

This aphorism brings faith in God to the foreground. According to certain masters, any undertaking in yoga, whether founded on faith or not, must come to it. Devotion is active and expresses itself in ritual and frequent prayers. Thoughts, speech, and actions are offered up to God.

This intensity of faith leads to contemplation and to the exceptional faculties that accompany it. These faculties are potential in every individual, though the ego hides them. Melting the ego and placing ourselves in the hands of a higher force reveals these faculties to us. Through them we discover that they are limited, and that those of the higher force are infinite.

The devotion presented in Chapter I is a way of attaining the yoga state. In the beginning of this chapter, devotion is presented as acceptance and nonattachment to the results of action—a daily attitude of being receptive to the deeper levels of being.

samādhisiddhirīśvarapraṇidhānāt
samādhi-siddhiḥ-īśvara-praṇidhānāt

Samādhi: contemplation. *Siddhiḥ:* power, accomplishment, realization. *Īśvara-praṇidhānāt:* through devotion to the Lord, positive behavior and the ritual act of devotion.

II.46

The posture is firm and soft.

Do I balance firmness with softness, strictness with ease, and stability with letting go?

If not, how can I develop these opposing, yet complementary, qualities in my daily life?

In my posture practice, is it best to:

- *not overdo things physically (sukha)?*
- *be strict about being present and conscious, not thinking of other things (sthira)?*

Does firmness in a posture practice include respect for a program, excessive effort, or strictly adhering to the program?

Does softness in a posture practice include adaptation, acceptance of limits, improvisation, or search for pleasure?

Are there limits to softness and firmness?

In the West, why has yoga practice focussed so heavily on the postural aspects?

What are the advantages and disadvantages of starting with postures?

Are postures more a means or an end?

What is the relationship between posture, discipline (II.43), self-reflection (II.44), and active devotion to God (II.45)?

In the West, the first approach to yoga is often through postures, for example, particular bodily positions such as standing, lying, inverting, sitting, and so on.

The Sanskrit word translated as "posture" (*āsanam*) is linked to the seated position itself, or to another posture or series of postures that lead up to it. It introduces other deeper components of yoga, such as breath control and meditation, and prepares the body and the mind for them.

The verbal root (*ās*) of *āsanam* is rich with meaning. It is the idea of being present in one's body—inhabiting, existing, and living in it. One acts without interruption or holds a position for a long while, maintaining it. There is also the idea of ritual.

Vigilance, or firmness, is physical stability, but, above all, presence, attention, and mental stillness. Complementary to that, softness and ease are the adaptation of posture to physical possibilities without force or excessive will. "It is attention without tension, loosening-up without slackness" (T.K.V. Desikachar.)

Firmness is the opposite of physical agitation (*aṅgamejayatva,* I.31), and ease is the opposite of suffering (*duḥkha,* I.31). Both firmness and softness are physical and mental. They form a whole that corresponds to the state of equilibrium (*sattva*), without agitation (*rajas*) or apathy (*tamas*). No yoga posture is real unless these two qualities are present together—they are constituents of the posture.

The posture is not just an externally codified position, but above all, is a subjective experience that brings the mind as well as the body into play. In everyday life, the posture firmly settles one's position because of these two complementary qualities: firmness over essential demands and softness in expressing them. Each personality emphasizes one or the other of these qualities, for the better development of each individual.

Briefly, the posture is to "be firmly established in a happy space" (Gérard Blitz).

sthirasukhamāsanam
sthira-sukham-āsanam

Sthira: firm, stable, without change, resolute, changeless. *Sukham:* easy, agreeable, comfortable, happy, prosperous, soft. *Āsanam:* yoga posture, seated, being seated, way of sitting, the camp, situation, place.

II.47

The posture is attained by pacification through correct effort and contemplating the infinite.

Is it harder for me to start practicing or to keep practicing? Or is my practice fairly effortless?

Does it take a certain headstrong will to reach a happy medium?

What distinctions can I draw between the expressions "firm and soft" (II.46) and "pacification through correct effort"?

How can I find concrete proof of the infinite in my postures?

Are there any dimensions within me that are not limited by birth or death?

Can observing the breath, which gives life to the body, help me become aware of my consciousness?

Does this aphorism mean:

- *that one never finishes exploring postures?*
- *that the practice of postures is lifelong?*

Why are relaxation and contemplation both necessary to attain the posture?

What is the link between seeking to unwind and seeking infinity?

Can it be said that practicing postures is praying, before, during, and after?

This aphorism gives us two means of mastering a posture. They are two aspects of one whole. Like ink and pen that together make writing possible, pacification through correct effort and contemplation of the infinite must both work, if either is to work.

Pacification through correct effort is the effort to practice regularly, to adapt this practice to one's possibilities and progress, to reduce tensions accumulated in the body, and lastly, to be relaxed and free in action. This is equilibrium and inner peace (*sattva*). Pacification (*śaithilya*) is the subtle level of respiration within the posture.

Contemplation of the infinite is awareness of an infinite dimension while the body remains still in a posture. How can we represent this infinite? On the one hand, the vital energy of breath lives in us; and on the other hand, consciousness contemplates the body made alive by the breath.

Contemplation also corresponds to "becoming aware of consciousness and breathing in the posture." The word "infinite" (*ananta*) illustrates, in itself, firmness and ease (II.46).

Acording to the Hindu tradition, *ananta* represents the serpent whose coils are a bed for the sleeping god *Viṣṇu,* and whose raised hood supports the universe. The serpent has to offer a soft and springy bed so as not to disturb Viṣṇu's meditation and, at the same time, furnish a sufficiently firm and stable support for the universe. Meditating on the infinite follows from studying and memorizing the *Yoga Sūtras.*

We can also perceive an infinite dimension in the innumerable postures, the variations, and the rhythm of breath. Everything in the techniques that pertains to a posture can lead to the graduations best suited to each one. The infinite also means that the posture is not an end in itself.

The term "contemplation" indicates entry into a more subtle dimension than the physical or psychic one; it is spirituality and prayer. In the Hindu tradition, a practical lesson of postures begins and ends with prayer. Some masters maintain that posture practice is prayer with the mind turned toward the infinite.

prayatnaśaithilyānantasamāpattibhyām
prayatna-śaithilya-ananta-samāpattibhyām

Prayatna: through correct effort, just, appropriate. *Śaithilya:* through relaxing, unwinding, pacification. *Ananta:* infinite. *Samāpattibhyām:* through meditation.

II.48

As a result, one is invulnerable to dualism.

Do people see me as hypersensitive or as insensitive and cold?

Does this aphorism mean that I should accept everything—become indifferent and tolerate everything?

What contradictions hamper me the most?

How can I reach equanimity and still retain real dynamism in life?

What is the difference between not complaining anymore and staying silent?

Is there a connection between disturbances raised by opposing pairs and ignorance (II.5)?

This third aphorism on posture describes what follows from the previous two. We live in a perpetually moving universe, where we have to undergo contradictory constraints that manifest as opposing pairs, such as cold and heat, immobility and mobility, success and setback, excess and lack (of work, for example), ambition and ability, love and hatred, birth and death, life and nothingness, change and conditioned habits.

Being torn between these poles is one of the great causes of suffering (II.15). These pairs of inevitable opposites bring tensions and conflicts in their wake. Being invulnerable does not mean being insensitive. It describes an appropriate reaction that makes it possible to avoid the avoidable and to better understand the inevitable. A correctly executed practice of postures, therefore, entails modifying reactions to outside influences by developing a judicious, adaptable attitude.

tataḥ dvandvānabhighātaḥ
tataḥ dvandva-anabhighātaḥ

Tataḥ: then, at this point. *Dvandva:* opposing pair or couple, duality, dualism. *Anabhighātaḥ:* invulnerability, undisturbed.

Once this is reached, breath control is the regulation of inhalation and exhalation.

How do I prepare myself to undertake prāṇāyāma regularly:

- *Can I remain seated long enough—that is, are my hips supple, my back strong, and my legs without "heaviness"?*
- *Is my respiration ample—that is, are my back and chest supple?*
- *Am I without physical or breath tensions, tics, or spasms linked to worry and stress?*
- *Am I free of unwanted impulses, such as burping, blinking, sneezing, yawning, and so on?*

If I think about something else while practicing breath control, am I outside the experience, regardless of how refined my technique is?

Although many yoga adepts are quite ready to practice postures every day, why do some find it so difficult to practice breath control regularly?

What psychological conditions are favorable if we want to harmonize breathing?

The three preceding aphorisms tell us that mastering postures is preliminary to breath control, which requires a still body and a calm mind. Mastering postures also alleviates:

- Symptoms that arise from obstacles in the personality (I.31), such as suffering, depression, restlessness, and irregular breathing.
- Spontaneous impulses (*vegas*) that manifest inner tension—blockage between *prāṇa* and *apāna*. They comprise four of the ten secondary breaths (*vāyus*) according to yoga: the "burp" (*nāga*), blinking (*kūrma*), sneezing (*kṛkara*), and yawning (*devadatta*). (*Gheraṇḍa-saṃhitā* V. 60).

In other words, the practice of breath control cannot be imposed. By mastering postures we develop at least the minimum physical well-being and mental peace that are necessary before approaching breath control. Immobility imposed by the will alone would give rise to tensions.

Most of the time, respiration is automatic and unconscious. It adapts itself to activities, thoughts, and moods, which often disturb it. Controlling the breath means leaving unconscious breathing behind to enter into conscious, regulated breathing. Such regulation of inhalation and exhalation favorably affects all of the organism's vital functions, that is, energy in all its forms in the body.

Breath regulation entails specific breath control techniques. Unconscious respiration needs to be cut (*chid*) to pass to conscious breathing.

The mastery of breath, manifestation of life, is a way of accessing the mastery of being as a whole. In fact, according to its etymology, the Sanskrit word *pra-ĀN-ā-YĀM-a* means to control, to master, to offer the different energies that give life to the body, pushing the experience to its utmost limits in order to reap the benefits. The *Bhagavad Gītā* defines *prāṇāyāma* as "...sacrificing the exhale in the inhale and the inhale in the exhale..." (B. G. IV.29).

tasminsatiśvāsapraśvāsayorgativicchedaḥ prāṇāyāmaḥ
tasmin-sati-śvāsa-praśvāsayoḥ-gati-vicchedaḥ prāṇāyāmaḥ

Tasmin: this, this latter (refers to āsanam, posture). *Sati:* being (verb). *Śvāsa:* disorderly, unharmonious, unconscious inhale. *Praśvāsayoḥ:* disorderly, unharmonious, unconscious exhale. *Gati:* of the movement. *Vicchedaḥ:* cessation, interruption. *Prāṇāyāmaḥ:* breath control.

The phases of breathing are exhalation, inhalation, and suspension. Observing them in space, time, and number, one is able to render breathing more harmonious in duration and subtlety.

Do I tend to breathe more air in or out? Do I spontaneously stop with my lungs full or empty?

Are these tendencies the result of a profession or a particular activity, such as swimming or playing a wind instrument?

Why is exhalation the primordial phase?

What do the different phases represent symbolically: inhalation, exhalation, full breath, empty breath, movement of breath (ventilation), and suspension of breath (apnea)?

Do I have sufficient inner focus for regular daily practice of prāṇāyāma?

Am I too vague, fairly strict, or overzealous in regulating the length of my breaths (inhalation, exhalation, and suspension)?

In my practice of prāṇāyāma over several days, am I consistent enough to avoid ups and downs?

Am I capable of maintaining about eighty percent of my real capacities, in order to avoid conflict and remain subtle (sukṣma)?

How will I know if I'm going too far with regard to length of time?

Can I develop the patience to wait for long-term results?

Can length of breath develop at the expense of subtlety, or subtlety at the expense of length? Which should I prefer?

If practicing prāṇāyāma has not increased sensitivity, attention, and patience, what conclusions should I draw?

This aphorism includes all the techniques contained in breath control:

- the way of breathing
- ways of regulating breathing
- the presence of two qualities and fundamental results

The phases of breathing are: exhalation (*bahya-vṛtti*), inhalation (*abhyantara-vṛtti*), suspension with lungs empty (*bahya-stambha-vṛtti*), suspension with lungs full (*abhyantara-stambha-vṛtti*) and, in intermediary states, suspension or techniques by degrees (*kramas*) (*stambha-vṛtti*). Exhalation, the movement of breathing out that expresses relaxation and giving, is the first to be addressed. Inhalation, or the movement of breathing in, was mentioned in aphorism I.31, which listed hurried breathing as a symptom of mental agitation.

The simple act of observing the breath makes it more even. Any overzealous intervention turns against the person practicing. This delicate observation passes in turn through the numerous breathing techniques, all of which concern space, time, and number, or some of these factors. This list covers the subtlest to the grossest.

- Space can designate the areas of the body where one feels the breath (thorax, abdomen, etc.), But above all, it corresponds to mental space—having disengaged one's mind and made time to practice breath control. It is also any element of concentration present in the mind, a sacred syllable (*mantra*), a concept, a master, or an image representing God. It is, therefore, either a perception or an image that the mind conceives or remembers.
- Time includes the duration appropriate to each movement of breath and the states of suspension, their proportions to each other, rhythms, and the total length of *prāṇāyāma* practice.
- Number applies to respirations and cycles.

The two final qualities indicate the aim, and the limits not to be exceeded. Breathing itself gets longer with regular, continuous practice over a long period. Subtlety intervenes on two levels. On the external level, the absence of disturbance is reflected in fluid, fine, regular respiration. On the internal level, a greater perceptual acuity appears, and one develops a sort of intimacy with oneself. There is no breath control where there is no length or subtlety.

bāhyābhyantarastambhavṛttirdeśakālasaṃkhyābhiḥ paridṛṣṭo dīrghasūkṣmaḥ
bāhya-ābhyantara-stambḥa-vṛttiḥ-deśa-kāla-saṃkhyābhiḥ paridṛṣṭaḥ dīrgha-sūkṣmaḥ

Bāhya: external. *Ābhyantara:* internal. *Stambḥa:* suspension. *Vṛttiḥ:* movement or type of operation. *Deśa:* space. *Kāla:* time. *Saṃkhyābhiḥ:* number, count. *Paridṛṣṭaḥ:* observed, mastered. *Dīrgha:* long. *Sūkṣmaḥ:* subtle, fine.

The fourth type of breath control transcends external or internal domains.

When I practice prāṇāyāma regularly, do I stay quiet afterward, observing the breath?

What mantra could I recite during prāṇāyāma, or what symbol could help me soar above mere technique?

Is this fourth type of prāṇāyāma a result or a means?

Is it an unforseeable state, or can one choose it?

Does this state chiefly concern the breath movements or movements of energy in the body as a whole?

What difference is there between this fourth type of breath control, concentration (dhāraṇa), and meditation (dhyāna, II.29)?

How can I avoid confusing certain pathological psychophysiological states in which breathing stops spontaneously with this fourth type of breath control?

This fourth type of breath control, as both result and means, goes beyond the phases of breathing. It can follow from daily practice of *prāṇāyāma.* For example, one must get into the habit of remaining seated in silence for a certain length of time after *prāṇāyāma,* and meditating on the breath at its source, which is the heart (*hṛdayam*). The use of mentally recited *mantras* during *prāṇāyāma* is a help. This fourth type of *prāṇāyāma* can also stem from a particular psychophysiological state or from divine grace. It is a state of accomplishment in breath control, of peace, and of deep calm not issuing from the will.

It soars above technique, being way above the material aspect, and reaches an indescribable, verbally intransmissible state.

bāhyābhyantaraviṣayākṣepī caturthaḥ
bāhya-ābhyantara-viṣaya-ākṣepī caturthaḥ

Bāhya: external, exterior. *Ābhyantara:* internal, interior. *Viṣaya:* domain, aspect, level. *Ākṣepī:* complete rejection, going beyond. *Caturthaḥ:* the fourth.

II.52

Then, all that veils clarity of perception is swept away.

Has regular practice of prāṇāyāma improved my lucidity and mental clarity?

Are observations of modified emotional states a good criterion for directing my prāṇāyāma practice?

What credit should I give to the opinions of others, the near and dear as well as strangers, with regard to appreciating my own mental clarity?

Does yoga exist without lucidity?

Is the state described here a definitive one?

What conclusions should I draw about continued practice of breath control?

Is this result also a means?

The body reaches equilibrium through posture practice. Through breath control, the mind itself reaches equilibrium. It is neither drowsy, nor slow in the uptake (*tamas*), nor in too much of a hurry, nor too impassioned (*rajas*) to be able to see clearly (*sattva*). There is better observation and understanding of the mind's reactions in a given situation.

The vision one has of oneself and the surrounding world becomes objective. It is undistorted by erroneous impulses such as ignorance, deformed or exaggerated consciousness of "I," passion, repulsion, or fear (II.3). A great lucidity, an unaccustomed sense of observation, and a quality of presence are very evident in one whose mental function has become transparent. The way is free to enter into the last three parts of yoga.

tataḥ kṣīyate prakāśāvaraṇam
tataḥ kṣīyate prakāśa-āvaraṇam

Tataḥ: then, there. *Kṣīyate:* is destroyed, reduced. *Prakāśa:* the light, clear perception. *Āvaraṇam:* the fact of covering, of hiding.

And thought becomes fit for concentration.

Is my concentration better since I started prāṇāyāma. If not, what should I do?

Does my concentration depend on which object I choose for it?

Is it easier for me to concentrate:

- *while actively doing something with my eyes open?*
- *on the breath or on a theme of meditation with my eyes closed?*

Is concentration an intentional and focused state, or a state where I let go due to breath control? Why?

Does this aphorism signify that a lack of concentration is one compelling reason to practice prāṇāyāma?

This aphorism presents concentration (the sixth limb of yoga) as the result of breath control (fourth limb). Why is the fifth limb only presented afterward?

According to Hindu tradition, thought (*manas*) is a component of the mind and one of the eleven sense organs (II.18). It functions automatically as a reflex, and if it lacks lucidity, the mind responds with ready-made answers.

The mind is prepared, through *prāṇāyāma,* to accede to a higher state—that of concentration, the sixth limb of yoga (II.29). The answers it gives will be new, inventive ones.

The word "concentration" means two things. On the one hand, authentic contemplation encompasses different objects. Otherwise, what appears to be concentration may be a state of attachment; the strong impression the first object makes would interfere during concentration on the second object. On the other hand, the state of concentration is a triple one, for it bears in it two developments: meditation (*dhyāna*) and contemplation (*samādhi*).

dhāraṇāsu ca yogyatā manasaḥ
dhāraṇāsu ca yogyatā manasaḥ

Dhāraṇāsu: in states of concentration. *Ca:* and. *Yogyatā:* aptitude, competence. *Manasaḥ:* of thought.

II.54

Withdrawal of the senses occurs when the sensory organs, independent of their particular objects, conform to the nature of mind.

Which objects "catch me" regularly?

With what organs of perception or action do I more usually attach myself to objects: hearing, touch, sight, taste, smell, speech, grasping or holding, locomotion, excretion, or generation?

Are the times after yoga practice or after rest or holidays conducive to discovering withdrawal of the senses?

Can putting aside a favorite, beautiful object, provisionally or definitely, help me to withdraw my sense organs?

Does isolation of any kind favor withdrawal of the senses?

Does real mastery of the sense organs mean one is no longer attracted to objects?

How can I avoid confusing this state with one of inhibiting desires (perception or action)?

What are the effects of frustration?

When one of the sense organs—hearing, for example—is focused on an object, can it be said that mastery of this sense organ would be:

- *not hearing?*
- *hearing, but choosing not to be disturbed or not to listen?*

What can such mastery bring to daily life and to our relationships with others?

What is the difference between this mastery of the senses, nonattachment (I.15), noncovetousness (II.39), and the means proposed in aphorism I.37?

Withdrawing at will from the sense organs follows the state of concentration. This is why the order of presenting these two limbs of yoga is reversed, as far as their numbering is concerned (II.29).

The mind, usually dispersed, depends on, is a slave even, to the sense organs themselves, forever attracted by outside solicitations.

The expression "sense organs" represents eleven elements, or senses. Besides the five senses of perception—hearing, touch, sight, taste, and smell—this mastery also includes the five senses of action—speech, sensory apprehension, locomotion, excretion, generation—and also the lower level of thought that coordinates these senses as a whole (*manas*).

The sense organs of perception are rightfully instruments that serve the mind, which is free to receive messages and control the activity of the sense organs of action.

Once we reach the state of concentration necessary for a more subtle research than the mere satisfaction of the senses, this capacity to accept or leave external situations in abeyance occurs spontaneously. Without frustration, it becomes possible to return home without flying straight to the radio, the television, the refrigerator, magazines, work, and so on. The choice is freely made. This stage is an excellent pointer to any personal evolution.

svaviṣayāsaṃprayoge cittasya svarūpānukāra ivendriyāṇām pratyāhāraḥ
sva-viṣaya-asaṃprayoge cittasya svarūpa-anukāraḥ iva indriyāṇām pratyāhāraḥ

Sva: his, her, proper, own. *Viṣaya:* domain, field of action. *Asaṃprayoge:* separation, dissociation. *Cittasya:* of the mind, spirit. *Svarūpa:* its peculiar, proper, own form, its nature. *Anukāraḥ:* resemblance, likeness, imitation, conformity. *Iva:* it is as if, in the same way as. *Indriyāṇām:* the (eleven) sense organs (of which thought...). *Pratyāhāraḥ:* withdrawal of the senses as far as objects are concerned.

II.55

It is then that the senses are perfectly mastered.

If there is no confrontation with the outer world, how shall I know if I have reached perfect mastery?

If mastery is to be authentic, does it have to embrace all the senses: the five senses of perception, the five organs of action, and coordinating thought?

How can I face the eventual loss of such mastery, once I have reached it?

What can be done with this extreme freedom?

This aphorism describes the results of the first limbs of yoga. This is a state of liberty, disentangled from all distraction (pleasure in seeing, in moving), without being in the thrall of erroneous impulses such as seeking after pleasure or passion.

Action is both correct and spontaneous, since the eleven sense organs have returned to their real function as instruments. An object no longer attracts a sense organ that, in turn, attracts the mind. Instead, the mind chooses freely and spontaneously to direct one of the sense organs toward an object. Such mastery does not mean indifference to other people. On the contrary, it links one to a great breadth of views and to a refined sensitivity, perfectly adapted to improving human relations.

Mastery of the sense organs is the basis of equilibrium and mental health, and therefore a major element of progress in yoga. Āyurvedic medicine points out that mental sickness and psychic disturbances have only one cause—bad management of desire.

tataḥ paramāvaśyatendriyāṇām
tataḥ paramā-vaśyatā-indriyāṇām

Tataḥ: then, from then on, there, as a result. *Paramā:* biggest, largest, highest or ultimate. *Vaśyatā:* mastery. *Indriyāṇām:* of the eleven sense organs (of which thought…).

CHAPTER III

Exceptional Faculties

vibhūtipādaḥ

EXCEPTIONAL FACULTIES

Do I have premonitions or other exceptional faculties? If so, how do I manage them?

How do I feel about these faculties and the supernatural?

According to Hindu tradition, the great age of these powers is a thing of the past. If we accept that, what can this chapter bring us?*

Chapter II introduced the eight limbs of the yoga of action as the most important way of fulfilling the intent of yoga, and addressed the first five limbs. Chapter III addresses the last three limbs and their goals. These three limbs are results rather than means—they are the flowering of yoga. In accomplishing them, one masters exceptional faculties. In opening these potentials one experiences not only their positive effects, but their dangers and limitations as well. With mastery of these accomplishments, yoga culminates in the state of liberation, which is the theme of Chapter IV.

The word *vibhūti,* translated here as exceptional faculties, is from the verb *vibhū,* which means "produce, is produced, manifests itself, is capable of." We can translate *vibhūti* in numerous ways: greatness of power, capacity, force, prosperity, success, dignity, rank, splendor, richness, riches, fortune, supernatural powers, ashes, and spiritual marks. Chapter III addresses these exceptional faculties and the last three limbs of yoga through answering the following questions:

III.1 to 3	What are the steps toward mastery?
III.4 to 8	What is mastery and how do we use it?
III.9 to 12	What are the different stages of transformation?
III.13 to 36	What do we mean by "exceptional faculties"?
III.37	What dangers do they present?
III.38 to 49	What are these exceptional faculties?
III.50 to 51	What should we avoid?
III.52 to 55	What is ultimate realization?

*The *Manava-dharma-astra* or Laws of Manou (ancient Hindu ethical moral code) distinguishes four ages. They correspond approximately to the four ages of the Greeks: *ktayuga* corresponds to the golden age, *tretyuga* corresponds to the silver age, *dvparayuga* corresponds to the brass age, *kaliyuga* corresponds to the iron age.

vibhūtipādaḥ
vibhūti-pādaḥ

Vibhūti: accomplishment, power. *Pādaḥ:* chapter, foot, quarter.

Concentration is focusing the mind on a particular point.

Do I find prolonged concentration easy or difficult?

Is it easier for me to concentrate on work, family life, leisure, or religious or spiritual endeavor?

How can I know whether I am concentrating or becoming attached (rāga, II.7)?

Is concentration a matter of work or of will?

Why must we stop running all over the place to attain a state of concentration?

After addressing the first five limbs of yoga, which relate to the body, respiration, and the sense organs, we now penetrate into yoga's mental, psychological, and spiritual dimensions: concentration (presented here), meditation, then contemplation, presented in the two following aphorisms.

Concentration is keeping the mind stable while directing it toward a particular object, whether surroundings are favorable or not. This "object," or space, on which the mind concentrates can belong to any sphere: a seen object, a concept, or an idea easily accessible or imponderable. For example, one might concentrate on a physical object, an object of research, a question, a problem, a relationship, or a metaphysical concept. Whatever the object, concentration on it must be free of excessive attachment, repulsion, or fear (II.7 to II.9).

In posture-based yoga, a first step toward concentration is observation of the body and breath.

deśabandhaścittasya dhāraṇā
deśa-bandhaḥ cittasya dhāraṇā

Deśa: place, space, particular point, territory, field of knowledge. *Bandhaḥ:* link, fixation, relationship. *Cittasya:* of the psyche, mind, intelligence, thought, sentiment, and emotion. *Dhāraṇā:* concentration, aptitude for directing mental activity.

III.2

Meditation is the uninterrupted flow of knowledge on this particular point.

Do I have the patience to wait for my concentration to open to a new and direct grasp of the object?

For me, what objects encourage meditation?

Can the feeling that something is not quite right be an object of meditation? Can meditation be a means of settling one's problems?

Does the aftermath of meditation reveal an authentic way of proceeding?

Why does learning something about myself during meditation enable me to appreciate the authenticity of that state?

Can meditation be taught?

With prolonged focus on one object, concentration becomes meditation, in which the grasp of the object is direct—instantaneous, new, and unforgettable. This interaction between subject and object leaves a deep impression that replaces understanding that is based on memory and the past.

Moving from mental dispersion to concentration is progressive. Passing from concentration (III.1) to meditation (III.2), however, is sudden and instantaneous, creating a break in the slowing curve of mental activity. Meditation is interplay between the inner and outer, expressed by a flash of knowledge on a chosen object.

The object of both concentration and meditation can be material, immaterial, known, or unknown (for example, the reason for difficulties in human relationships). In other texts, the word *dhyāna* assumes the meaning of reflection or even of prayer, the first cause of all being God.

tatra pratyayaikatānatā dhyānam
tatra pratyaya-ekatānatā dhyānam

Tatra: there, in that case, such a case. *Pratyaya:* experience, contents of the mind. *Ekatānatā:* fixed on one point during a certain time. *Dhyānam:* meditation, aptitude for unfallibly developing interactions with what we try to understand.

When the object of meditation alone shines in the mind, as though the mind is emptied of its own form—that is contemplation.

How does contemplation with eyes closed prepare me for contemplation in action, with my eyes open?

Is contemplation an act of will or surrender?

Does contemplation require letting a higher dimension work within me?

Does contemplation imply losing all notion of time and space?

How does regular, repeated experience of contemplation change my personality?

What are the pitfalls of the way of contemplation?

Why does Patañjali address the first five limbs in one chapter and these last three limbs in another?

Contemplation, a state often desired, sought after, and sometimes feared, prolongs concentration and meditation.

In Chapter I, Patañjali mentioned that in contemplation, all that remains of an object is its essence. Other ways of apprehending an object, for example, its name or shape, have vanished.

Understanding of the object shines brightly in the mind, to the point where it eclipses reflective consciousness, just as daylight eclipses the light of the stars in the sky. In other words, the grasp of the object is so strong that perception of one's own personality seems to have vanished. The reality of the object is so intense we forget ourselves. This is a provisional state.

tadevārthamātranirbhāsaṃ svarūpaśūnyamiva samādhiḥ
tad-eva artha-mātra-nirbhāsaṃ svarūpa-śūnyam-iva samādhiḥ

Tad: that (with reference to *dhyāna*). *Eva*: correctly, precisely. *Artha:* essence, signification, aim, exact nature of. *Mātra:* only, that alone, measure of. *Nirbhāsam:* manifestation, apparition, brilliance. *Svarūpa:* its own shape. *Śūnyam:* emptiness, void, desert. *Iva:* as if, so to speak. *Samādhiḥ:* contemplation, complete fusion, integration with an object of meditation.

III.4

Perfect mastery is prolonged focus on one object through sustained states of concentration, meditation, and contemplation.

Am I able to choose a focus in yoga—postures, breathing techniques, certain texts, mantras, or certain concepts (nonviolence, etc.)—and stay with it for several years?

Which ones suit my personality, my tastes, or my possibilities?

In the long run, how can this mastery change my personality, and what dangers are likely?

The teacher, T. Krishnamacharya, states that yoga is "perfect mastery of the body, the breath, the senses, and the mind" (Śarīra-prāṇa-indriya-mano saṃyamaḥ yogaḥ). What can I conclude from this?

What is the difference between mastery of a certain field, such as science, and the mastery presented here?

Perfect mastery (*saṃyama*) is successive passage through sustained states of concentration, meditation, and contemplation on one object to reach an almost complete and exhaustive understanding of it.

This aphorism opens the way to the powers introduced in this chapter, most of which are obtained through this perfect mastery.

This meaning of the Sanskrit word saṃyama—perfect mastery—is different from the meaning it assumes in other texts where its meaning is closer to renunciation, religious vow, or control of the senses (*Bhagavad Gītā* II.61; IV.26 and IV.27). These different interpretations are not contradictory. To keep the mind focused on one and the same object over time demands total investment of the being and restriction of incursions into other fields. However, this engagement must be free from passion or it becomes blind and sectarian. Perfect mastery, therefore, implies discernment, that is, nonattachment to the faculties acquired.

trayamekatra saṃyamaḥ
trayam-ekatra saṃyamaḥ

Trayam: triad, being three. *Ekatra:* on one point. *Saṃyamaḥ:* perfect mastery, renunciation, control, religious vow, act of penitence.

The light of the highest knowledge comes from acquisition of this perfect mastery.

What is the difference between appreciating someone for excellence in a certain field and appreciating someone personally?

What is the wisdom of such recognition?

Can the light of knowledge of one object also be applied to other objects?

How does one prevent or remedy errors resulting from poor integration of this mastery, for example, feeling one's path or field is superior to all others?

The establishment of perfect mastery enables one to attain certain results: knowledge of the object of endeavor and wisdom acquired from mastery. In other words, one first masters the object, and thereafter, masters mastery itself.

Devoting oneself to the practice of breath control (*prāṇāyāma*) over several years, for example, can one day bring an extraordinary grasp of this breath that gives us life—intransmissible in words as an experience, except perhaps in poetry. Such exceptional knowledge can lead one to consider any other approach to yoga as inferior. But we must still accept that there are other ways of approach for other people.

It goes without saying that we must attain knowledge before we can leave it behind.

tajjayātprajñālokaḥ
tad-jayāt-prajñā-lokaḥ

Tad: that (relates to sayama). *Jayāt:* through victory, conquest, triumph. *Prajñā:* higher knowledge, wisdom. *Lokaḥ* light.

III.6

This perfect mastery is necessary to the stages that remain.

How can I reinvest my capacities in my practice?

Can I determine my own level? If not, what should I do?

How can I avoid copying someone who starts from a level higher than my own?

Yoga brings ease, self-confidence, and skill. How can we avoid giving these over to money, power, or honors?

Whatever level I reach, how can I stay in touch with beginners to be able to give them what they need?

Is my daily practice of yoga based on my own needs, or on those of my students? What should I conclude from this?

That Patañjali should speak of stages clearly underlines that evolution unfolds step by step, bringing the need for intermediary objectives and different methods at each stage. For some, acquired capacities are stepping-stones to a new stage. For others, watching another's evolution can help them understand their own possibilities and respect their own demands and needs. Yoga should be adapted to the individual and not the individual to yoga. The light thrown by a guide is important in the choice of objectives.

To conclude, the word *viniyoga* means evolution—adapting the means to each stage, intelligent use of acquired capacities, and transmission as an offering, all without seeking personal gain. As Śri T.K.V. Desikachar says: "The spirit of *viniyoga* is starting from where one finds oneself. As everybody is different and changes from time to time, there can be no common starting point, and ready-made answers are useless. The present situation must be examined and the habitually established status must be reexamined."

tasya bhūmiṣu viniyogaḥ
tasya bhūmiṣu viniyogaḥ

Tasya: of this. *Bhūmiṣu:* stage, landing, platform, step. *Viniyogaḥ:* employing, using, applying, disposing, abandoning.

The last three limbs of yoga are more internal than the first five.

Which grouping (below) of the eight limbs favors my evolution?

How can I assess which of my students need to practice further with the first five limbs and which are ready to approach the last three limbs?

Are a calm, peaceful, collected attitude and a certain ease in life good criteria for assessment? What other criteria might be good?

Does engagement in the last three limbs imply never returning to the first five?

If one is engaged in a method based primarily in the last three limbs, is it necessary to have passed through the first five before handing it on?

Do the first five limbs belong to the sphere of doing, and the last three to the sphere of being? Do the first five belong to the way of approach and the last three to results? Why is this, and what can I conclude?

How can I prevent a more inward endeavor from cutting me off from external realities?

This and the following aphorism expand on and explain the preceding one, which introduced the notion of stages: *bhūmi* (III.6). The eight limbs of yoga addressed in Chapter II can be divided into two groups.

In the first group are:

- *yama:* principles of respect with regard to others and self
- *niyama:* personal principles of positive action
- *āsana:* posture
- *prāṇāyāma:* breath control
- *pratyāhāra:* withdrawing oneself at will from the sense organs of perception, action, and monitoring

In the second group are:

- *dhāraṇā,* concentration
- *dhyāna,* meditation
- *samādhi,* contemplation

According to the commentary to aphorism II.29, the first five limbs concern the individual's relationship with the external world and the physical and energetic levels of human being.

Compared with the first five, the last three limbs are said to be concerned with the inner dimension, that is, the subtle universe, the psyche, thought, and consciousness. This notion corresponds to the living experience of one who progressively reaches greater consciousness and enters deeper and deeper into his or her own being.

Numerous concrete signs can indicate levels attained in the first group: strength, suppleness, breathing rhythm, speech, and so on. Levels reached in the second group, however, are less obvious, because these three limbs correspond to the more hidden, secret universe of consciousness.

Different teachings stem from this. For example, some teach the need for a structured personality before entering on the path of meditation. Just as valid is letting the degree of a person's inwardness or outwardness guide the choice of an aim. Lastly, Patañjali introduces the limbs as relative to each other, a notion that he insists on in the next aphorism.

trayamantaraṅgaṃ pūrvebhyaḥ
trayam-antar-aṅgaṃ pūrvebhyaḥ

Trayam: triad, triple, group of three (further reference to *dhāraṇā, dhyāna, samādhi*). *Antar:* internal, within, in the middle, inside. *Aṅgaṃ:* member, limb, part. *Pūrvebhyaḥ:* anterior, that which goes before, preceding.

These last three limbs must themselves be seen as external compared to contemplation without a seed.

What can consciousness of relativity teach me about my own and others' achievement and success?

Stages being relative, can I ever think I have arrived?

"Contemplation without a seed" is spontaneous, whereas "contemplation with a seed" has successive degrees. Can any state of contemplation that occurs spontaneously be considered more internal, and therefore, superior? What can I conclude from this?

In this aphorism, Patañjali places relative values on both groups of the limbs of yoga. The first five limbs are external compared to last three, which are internal and directly related to consciousness. These last three limbs, including contemplation, however, are less internal than the ultimate contemplation without a seed presented at the end of Chapter I. In this ultimate state of open availability, the mind instantaneously grasps everything.

The notion of "internal" or "external" applied to the limbs of yoga is, therefore, that each is quite relative to the limbs before and after it. The limbs are equally relative from one person to another. There is no overall universal scale of values for themes of inquiry or levels attained. As perfect mastery is based on individual needs and capacities, all is relative.

It can be said that the inward path never ends, as the Indian proverb quoted early in this book gives us to understand: "You can plumb the depths of a well, but the depths of the mind are unfathomable."

tadapi bahiraṅgaṁ nirbījasya
tad-api bahiḥ-aṅgaṁ nirbījasya

Tad: this, this latter (the triad). *Api:* even, same, as well. *Bahiḥ:* external. *Aṅgam:* the limb, member. *Nirbījasya:* contemplation without seed (*samādhi:* understood, cf. I.51).

III.9

When after a moment of stability, the mind ceases its fluctuation and remains naturally quiet, it begins its transformation to stability.

On leaving a special place or time of practice (religious retreat, etc.) do I remain at peace? If not, why?

What can I do to draw closer to that state and not fall back again?

As yoga replaces the usual habits that cause suffering (II.15) with the habit of liberating attitudes (I.50, I.51, III.9):

- *What are the primary habits that condition my existence?*
- *Which habits are harmful and what should replace them?*
- *Which habits are favorable and how do I reinforce them?*

Regular experience of meditative and contemplative states leads to a deep transformation of the personality that occurs in three stages. This and the following three aphorisms address this transformation.

The first stage, described here, is a permanent state of stability in which one engaged in activity keeps an even mind.

The mind, projected outward and slipping out of control, gives rise to similar situations: dispersion draws with it a return to dispersion. It is the same with stability and peace. There comes a day when peaceful habits—moments of stability—carry the day against habits of dispersion. A natural tendency then appears: the mind returns to equilibrium at every transitory period. This change is a transformation to stability.

vyutthānanirodhasaṃskārayorabhibhavaprādurbhāvau nirodhakṣaṇacittānvayo nirodhapariṇāmaḥ
vyutthāna-nirodha-saṃskārayoḥ abhibhava-prādurbhāvau nirodha-kṣaṇa-citta -anvayaḥ nirodha-pariṇāmaḥ

Vyutthāna: mental fluctuation. *Nirodha:* cessation. *Saṃskāra:* mental permeation. *Abhibhava:* disappearance. *Prādurbhāvau:* manifestation. *Kṣaṇa:* instant. *Citta:* the psyche, mind, thought. *Anvaya:* following. *Pariṇāmaḥ:* change, mutation, transformation.

This peaceful flow within the mind is born of its own latent impressions.

Do I naturally remain positive in all circumstances?

How does a positive attitude help in the teaching of yoga?

What are the effects of discovering that, on the whole, our behavior is repetitive, even when we think it is spontaneous?

Does yoga suppress habits or does it replace painful ones with stable ones?

Can replacing bad habits with good ones culminate in total spontaneity?

Does this aphorism mean that, at this peaceful level, all effort is useless and vigilance is no longer necessary?

Our thoughts, our speech, and our behavior are usually repetitive. Habits such as taste and the way we talk and dress influence our evolution.

There are two sorts of opposing habits: negative ones, which in the long run, drag us into suffering (II.5) and positive habits, which bring us nearer the yoga state.

The day dawns when habits of mental peace and positive thought create a dynamic, full of its own momentum, that ends the return to negative habits.

tasya praśāntavāhitā saṃskārāt
tasya praśānta-vāhitā saṃskārāt

Tasya: of this, this latter. *Praśānta*: appeased, calm, tranquil. *Vāhitā:* flow, current, outflow. *Saṃskārāt:* because of impregnation, permeation, of latency, of mental impression.

III.11

In the transformation to contemplation, distraction vanishes and the mind becomes focused.

Am I often centered on one activity or one thought?

Does this depend on the type of activity (professional, family, yoga or religious practice, etc.)? What should I conclude?

How can I differentiate between a schizoid tendency and the state described in this aphorism?

How can I keep an open mind and be attentive to others, yet at the same time, remain focused on one point?

A second transformation of the personality can come about after the first one. It is marked by the natural way in which the mind centers on one thing to apprehend it better, even though at each moment there are numerous possible choices. This stability is not the result of attachment or excessive passion (II.7).

This state clarifies the definition of yoga given in aphorisms 1, 2, 3 and 4 in this chapter. The mind no longer fluctuates. If it did, the mind engaged in one activity would still be looking for another, like an insatiable viewer of television who is always switching channels.

According to some scientific observations, the mind can grasp only one thing at a time, passing extremely quickly from one to another. This gives an impression of simultaneity, and the illusion of movement as in a film. A focused mind is a natural state that recenters all energies, allowing great acuteness in observation as well as in action. This state gives optimal force to the mental function, like a laser beam.

sarvārthataikāgratayoḥ kṣayodayau cittasya samādhipariṇāmaḥ
sarvārthatā-ekāgratayoḥ kṣaya-udayau cittasya
samādhi-pariṇāmaḥ

Sarvārthatā: multidirectional, multiplicity of objects. *Ekāgratayoḥ:* in one direction, focused. *Kṣaya:* destruction, loss, diminishing. *Udayau:* emerging, rising, appearance. *Cittasya:* of the psyche, mind, thought. *Samādhi:* contemplation, union. *Pariṇāma:* transformation, mutation.

Following contemplation is transformation to one-pointedness, in which one experiences with equanimity both mental peace and the return to a less coherent former state.

Am I thrown off balance by my failures?

If so, can I change this?

How can I strive toward a unique aim, yet be detached from the result?

What part do success and the lack of it play in life?

How do I differentiate between the exceptional state presented in this aphorism and overblown self-satisfaction?

How can being deeply anchored in mental peace, free of fluctuations, affect concrete aspects of life, such as success or lack of it, age, or health?

Even when one is established in contemplation (III.11) and the mind is at peace and focused, sickness may still blow one off course through flashbacks to former mental states.

This aphorism describes a state in which we no longer pass judgment, but fully accept our own reality, whatever it may be. At this point, success, or the lack of it, no longer directly influences the direction we choose. That does not mean it is an immobile state free of questioning, but a state that perpetually evolves toward a stable course.

The premature use of this teaching could lead to self-complacency; for example, not taking responsibility for one's negative attitude and expecting others to take it or leave it. To conclude, this state appears as the aftermath of preceding states. It means total acceptance of one's personality.

tataḥ punaḥ śāntoditau tulyapratyayau cittasyaikāgratāpariṇāma
tataḥ punaḥ śānta-uditau tulya-pratyayau
cittasya ekāgraāt-pariṇāma

Tataḥ: thereafter, there. *Punaḥ:* again, once more. *Śānta*: appeasement. *Uditau:* manifestation, appearance. *Tulya:* identical, similar. *Pratyayau:* mental experience. *Cittasya:* of the psyche, mind, and thought. *Ekāgratā:* one-pointedness, focusing. *Pariṇāmaḥ:* transformation, mutation.

The evolution of fundamental tendencies, of relationship to time, and of situations, all of which intervene in the physical constitution and the organs of perception and action, is thus explained.

Until now, how have my physical form and my behavior evolved?

Observing them enables me to evaluate the way I do yoga. What should I do if:

- *nothing seems to have changed?*
- *I change too quickly, for example, for my partner?*
- *the direction evolution takes is unfavorable?*

Why is it that changing my situation is more conducive to evolution than rearranging my time or priorites?

Is it always easy to change the situation in which one is involved?

What does time have to do with changing a given situation?

Is changing too often a flight from reality?

How do I know when to take responsibility for a situation and when to leave it alone?

With appearances, everything changes. The paper I am reading was once a tree and one day will be recycled or burned. My gold ring was once ore in the soil. What will it become in the hands of my great grandchildren?

It is the same with our physical forms and psyches, which change constantly within the fields of our potentials.

Three successive, specific states have been presented: the transformations toward stability, contemplation, and one-pointedness. These take place on two levels: first, within what really changes, and second, within the fields in which the changes occur.

Three types of reality can change: fundamental tendencies, relation to time, and situation:

- Fundamental tendencies include personal values—being a believer or not, for example.
- Temporal characteristics include age, which must be accepted, and the perception and allocation of time, which can be modified.
- Situation includes family, social, and professional situations, as well as quality of mind, which can evolve from inertia to activity to equilibrium (see constituent qualities of nature, *guṇa,* II.18).

Such changes appear in one's body and in one's relationship with the surroundings. In this way, health and physical form and possibilities evolve along with the way one perceives the world, acts, thinks, and behaves.

The possibility of evolution is greater with changes of situation, moderate with regard to time, and feeble in terms of our values. It is by changing a situation that one can better employ one's time and, in the end, modify one's priorities and scale of values.

etena bhūtendriyeṣu dharmalakṣaṇāvasthāpariṇāmā vyākhāyāt
etena bhūta-indriyeṣu dharma-lakṣaṇa-avasthā-pariṇāmāḥ vyākhāyāt

Etena: in, it follows that. *Bhūta:* in the basic elements (earth, water, fire, air, and ether). *Indryeṣu:* in the organs of perception and action. *Dharma:* the law of the individual; values. *Lakṣaṇa:* time, period, epoch. *Avasthā:* situation, condition, state, state of mind. *Pariṇāmāḥ:* transformation, change, mutation. *Vyākhyātāḥ:* being explained.

III.14

One substratum contains past, present, and future characteristics.

How can I better understand my inner nature—the unchangeable and the changeable in me?

How can this discovery help me learn of my own destiny and another's?

What influence does it have on my respect for another?

This aphorism sets out the limits of change. Every element takes on numerous forms, for example, water can be a solid (ice), liquid, or gas (steam), depending on temperature. At a given moment, a single form manifests, ice for example, when it is cold. In the same way, each of us carries a multitude of gifts within—qualities that may or may not show themselves, depending on the situation. Our capacities may be categorized in three ways: those that have been shown—the past; those that are showing—the present; and those still hidden away—the future.

Our changes are limited by a basic substratum, characteristic of our inner nature, that resists all outside influence. Our personalites rest on this substratum and our influence on another stops here. The martyr, for example, prefers death to denial of his or her beliefs.

According to the teaching of Patañjali's yoga, such a substratum also exists in "nature," *prakṛti* (original matter)—the fingerprint, for example. The support for the individual spiritual entity is *puruṣa* (consciousness, witness of transformations).

In short, the universe is divided into two parts: change (*pariṇama vāda*) and being (*sat vāda*). This perception is the foundation of yoga teaching. Suffering is reduced by adaptation to change. But, trying to pull others outside the limits of their possibilities will make their suffering worse or make them leave.

śāntoditavyapadeśyadharmānupātī dharmī
śānta-udita-avyapadeśya-dharma-anupātī dharm

Śānta: the past, pacified. *Udita:* the present, spring up, emerged. *Avyapadeśya:* the future. *Dharma:* the law, scale of values. *Anupātī:* that comes after. *Dharmī:* basic characteristics, the essential, the support.

Different methods produce different changes.

What methods best suit my temperament and best serve my evolution?

How can I avoid trying to force others to follow my way when it does not suit them?

What are the advantages and disadvantages of imitation in teaching and learning yoga?

Having introduced the different possibilities of evolution, Patañjali presents the idea of method—a way of attaining things. Many methods exist for changing situations, and the order of the degrees of apprenticeship is adaptable. To acquire a certain level in a foreign language, for example, one might take classes, individual lessons, or a correspondence course, or one might stay in the country where the language is spoken. The rate of learning differs according to the method used.

The method must also suit a student's aptitudes and temperament. For example, a gregarious person who is not so fond of books and solitude would learn more with a maximum of human contact and, therefore, might prefer to spend time with native speakers of the language.

On another level, this aphorism reconsiders the idea that the chosen path is direct or progressive, with intermediary stages according to one's temperament (I.22). Other factors that determine the method of approach are will power, capacity for sustained effort, vital energy, adaptability, constancy, and inner peace. Knowing someone's own temperament and how it relates to method enables a teacher to avoid drawing pupils of another temperament on paths that lead nowhere. This is the mark of the real guide (*guru*).

kramānyatvaṃ pariṇāmānyatve hetuḥ
krama-anyatvaṃ pariṇāma-anyatve hetuḥ

Krama: progression, method, way of proceeding. *Anyatvam:* difference, diversity. *Pariṇāma:* transformation, change. *Anyatve:* difference, diversity. *Hetuḥ:* cause.

III.16

Knowledge of the past and the future proceeds from the mastery of threefold evolution: fundamental, temporal, and situational.

How do I feel about paths I have taken in the past?

Am I clear about my present situation, my values, and how I spend my time?

How can I foresee ongoing and future inflections of my past evolution?

How important is this aphorism for those whose profession orients and advises others in their evolution?

Why and to what extent is discretion important when this power appears?

Is an excess of self-analysis possible? What would its consequences be?

Frequent concentration, meditation, and contemplation on one object has, thus far, been the theme of this chapter. This allows us to evolve through three stages before realizing extraordinary faculties. Such faculties have two aspects: They can be a way of growth or a decided pitfall. Patañjali devotes the end of this chapter to extraordinary faculties and introduces the first aspect here.

Through regular exploration, followed by evolution of our deep-seated tendencies and relationships to time and situations, we can develop knowledge of the past and the future.

It may seem surprising that being informed about one's past should be presented as an exceptional result, for where is the person who does not know his or her own past? But, Patañjali is speaking here about the causes that determine our choices, the directions taken, and past facts.

By discovering the thread that links past events to each other and to deep-seated tendencies in our personality, we are better able to see possible orientations of the future and to let go of utopian dreams. This gives us the opportunity of firmly making choices for certain appropriate options.

Who does not dream of knowing his or her future, drifting toward astrologers and fortunetellers? The method here is more rational. After such an undertaking ourselves, we can understand another's past and future.

Someone who can thus better direct his or her own future can also help others in judiciously choosing objectives and methods (III.15). Surely, the great masters, who understand their past mistakes, give others insight on the right way to proceed in order to avoid future pitfalls.

pariṇāmatrayasaṃyamādatītāngatajñānam
pariṇāma-traya-saṃyamāt-atīta-angata-jñānam

Pariṇāma: change, modification, mutation, transformation. *Traya:* triad, being triple, threefold. *Saṃyamāt:* because of perfect mastery, renunciation, control, religious vow, act of penitence. *Atīta:* that that is past, dead, or gone. *Anāgata:* the future, that has not yet happened. *Jñānam:* knowledge.

III.17

Interaction among words, their objects, and one's image or idea engenders confusion. Mastering distinction among them allows understanding of the sounds that creatures make.

Does what I say take into account what I think consciously or unconsciously?

If not, how can I close the gap?

To what extent can paying attention to others' remarks give us insight into the real meaning of our speech?

Is there a link between this aphorism and the psychoanalyist's "floating attention?"

Does this aphorism imply that our inablility to understand what others say comes from us?

What do my tone of voice and my lapses really mean?

In our time, when communication is so important, this aphorism is singularly appropriate. Before becoming living proof of "the gift of tongues" (attained by the Apostles at Whitsuntide according to the Gospels), however, the first stage is to understand what we are actually saying.

Very often there is a gap between the words we use and what these words really mean, because our inner and outer experiences color them. Something that sounds like a compliment might really be expressing jealousy that the speaker seeks to hide even from him- or herself.

The first stage, then, is prolonged observation of the possible gap between our own words and what we are really saying, given our situations, our experiences, and our emotional and mental states. It is a matter of knowing what we say, why we say it, and in what circumstances we say it.

Once we are able to do this for ourselves, it becomes possible to understand what others are saying better than they themselves do. Among other things, differences related to sex, temperament, and social or cultural background, make communication difficult. Careful expression and observation enables us to be understood outside our own environment—for example, to leave colloquial or special uses of language, such as jargon, behind.

One means of attaining this faculty in yoga's oral tradition is chanted repetition. Having to reproduce exactly what one hears the teacher say, little by little, each student discovers his or her own characteristics and meaning.

Since psychoanalysis is founded on observation and decoding of speech, can we say that it attempts something similar to what this aphorism is saying?

The accord between thought and word is so important and so difficult to achieve that the chief religions present God as truth, or veracity.

śabdārthapratyayānāmitaretarādhyāsātsaṅkarastat-
pravibhāgasaṃyamātsarvabhūtarutajñānam
śabd-ārtha-pratyayānām-itaretarādhyāsāt-saṅkaraḥ-tat-pravibhāga-
saṃyamāt sarva bhūta-ruta-jñānam

Śabda: word, verb, speech, sound. Artha: meaning, essence, aim. Pratyayānām: experience, contents of the mind. Itaretara: one or the other, mutual. Adhyāsāt: because of being falsely attributed to. Saṅkaraḥ: confusion, mixture. Tat: that. Pravibhāga: distinction, separation, division. Saṃyamāt: because of, due to perfect mastery, renunciation, control, religious vow, act of penitence. Sarva: all. Bhūta: creature, element. Ruta: cry, chant, sound in general. Jñānam: knowledge.

III.18

Knowledge about the origins of previous stages appears when we gain insight into our own conditioning.

Do I often fall into the same situations, making the same false starts?

Do my most ingrained habits stem from heredity, education, or imitation of a parent, friend, or other person?

Which of my difficulties can block the freedom to change? Which qualities might enhance it?

Is there a connection between this aphorism and psychoanalysis?

With this aphorism, Patañjali proposes we look our own conditioning squarely in the eye: atavistic, hereditary, family, educational, social, professional, and so on. But how can we do so? Among other possibilities, we might simply try something new—a new way of doing something or a different culture. A westerner using chopsticks for the first time, for example, might be surprised by the issues it raises.

All behavior originates within a specific historical and sociocultural context. The same sort of behavior can go on seemingly forever, even when surroundings have changed. Beginning most of our responses with "no," as a result of being in aggressive or offensive surroundings, can go on for years after we've moved to more favorable ones. Becoming conscious of our negative expressions leads to the discovery of their origins and can liberate us from them.

To look our habits straight in the eye, we might need to change our activities, to stop, or to change place or surroundings. Knowing more about our origins enables us to make new choices and get a fresh start.

saṃskārasākṣtkaraṇātpūrvajātijñānam
saṃskāra-sktkṣāaraṇāt-pūrva-jāti-jñānam

Saṃskāra: conditioning. *Sākṣātkaraṇāt:* because one has something under one's nose, under one's gaze, through perception. *Pūrva:* anterior, beforehand. *Jāti:* birth, caste. *Jñānam:* knowledge.

Knowing what another is thinking comes from perfect mastery of the mind's contents.

Do I know where my thoughts come from or how they connect with my emotions, even if the emotions are blocked or unconscious? What is the role of thoughts and how do outside influences affect them?

How can I foster such consciousness?

To what extent must we further develop discretion as this faculty awakens,?

How can I explore my own consciousness sufficiently, and at the same time, free myself from it enough to observe another's?

Does the awakening of this faculty depend on predominance of one of the three constituent qualities of nature (guṇas)?

Patañjali proposes a way of reading another's thoughts, something many people would like to do. The means he advises is continual observation, until one has mastered the contents of the mind. One must first know oneself and master the mind before having a flash of blinding intuition into another person's thoughts. In the psychoanalytic sense of the term, this is becoming conscious of projection.

Before we examine another persons mind, therefore, we must become conscious of the factors that condition us. We must first know and accept ourselves, so that we are sufficiently calm. Then, the image of the other can be reflected on the calm surface of our mind. When we are calm and listening, and accustomed to seeing the influence of fear on our own attitudes, breathing patterns, and facial expressions, we will be able to feel another's fear. If we have not gotten over our own fears, we are likely to see only our own fear in another. This is the same for all human feelings.

pratyayasya paracittajñānam
pratyayasya para-citta-jñānam

Pratyayasyā: of the mind's contents. *Para:* other, different, ultimate. *Citta:* psyche, mind, intelligence, thought, sentiment, emotion. *Jñānam:* knowledge.

III.20

The origin of another's thought is not grasped, because it cannot be observed.

How can I let go of wanting to interpret another's thoughts?

What are the likely risks of these interpretations?

What are the ramifications of each of us having our own "secret garden?"

Is it ever wise to draw conclusions about the causes of a persons illness, particularly if the illness is psychological?

Having proposed in the preceding aphorism the mind-reading power so many people dream of, Patañjali here points out the limitations. If one is clear about the contents of one's own mind, it becomes possible to feel the sentiments that animate another. This phenomenon, arising in a state of perfect concentration, implies that only one object shows itself in the observer's sphere of consciousness. It becomes impossible, therefore, to gain access to the circumstances, objects, or events that have brought about the other's mental state, because only one perception is possible at a time.

For example, if we are speaking with someone and we sense something of their psychological complexion or have flashes of insight or images that reinforce this intuition, how can we be sure where they come from? There are so many possibilities: the speaker is a professional psychologist, or has just been seen by a psychologist, or again, has just been reading a book on psychology that colors his or her mental state, and so on.

This aphorism emphasizes the possible danger in interpreting one's impressions too quickly, so great is the risk of mistakes. Patañjali is extremely wary in this sphere; however, other systems of thought affirm that a great master can also understand the causes of another's thought.

na ca tatsālambanaṃ tasyāviṣayībhūtatvāt
na ca tat-sālambanaṃ tasya-aviṣayī-bhūtatvāt

Na: no. *Ca:* and. *Tat:* that. *Sālambanam:* leaning on. *Tasya:* of that. *Aviṣayī:* without object. *Bhūtatvāt:* because of nature.

Invisibility comes from perfect mastery of physical appearance, which allows one to dissociate the observer's gaze from one's own emanations.

Do I draw attention to myself or pass unnoticed?

What qualities should I develop in order to pass unnoticed or for people to notice me more?

When one takes steps never to be seen, is it a show of this power, or fear of being asked to participate?

It is possible to attract more or less attention. One can disappear, like a chameleon, by imitating the dress, behavior, and personality of others, or stand out by being different. Unless there is interest in the thing seen, there is no perception. Interaction between the eye and the object registers the view, but the mind has to send out its intention to perceive the image. A person can attract another's eye to a greater or lesser extent by playing on the spectator's interest. This faculty also includes the other senses; one might hear, feel, touch, or taste something more or less.

At a higher level, it is possible to become completely invisible. The way of proceeding is the same: Be fully conscious of your own body, become aware of how others see it, and influence that relationship.

kāyarūpasaṃyamāttadgrāhyaśaktistambhe
cakṣuḥprakāśasaṃprayoge'ntardhānam
kāya-rūpa-saṃyamāt-tad.-grāhya-śakti-stambhe
cakṣuḥ-prakāśa-asaṃprayoge-antardhānam

Kāya: body. *Rūpa:* shape. *Saṃyamāt:* due to perfect mastery. *Tad:* that. *Grāhya:* can be grasped. *Śakti:* power. *Stambhe:* suppression. *Caku:* eye. *Praka:* light, appearing. *Asaṃprayoge:* disconnection. *Antardhānam:* disappearance.

III.22

Perfect mastery of slow and rapid evolution of actions brings knowledge of the time and circumstances of one's own death. This is also known through premonition.

How can I observe the evolution of my actions and their results?

How can this aphorism help me to choose objectives?

Am I more likely to use this observation-based method, or, am I fortunate enough to have well-founded premonitions?

How can anticipating certain phenomena change the way I live?

Some actions have an immediate result, such as displacing a rock. Others are slower, planting a tree, for example. Beyond these elementary examples, observing our actions calls for long-term experience. The rhythm of transformation depends as much on the mental attitudes, motives, and objectives of the person acting as it does on the type of action itself. Such discernment helps a teacher choose objectives for a student and list them according to the chances of their success. Choosing a rapidly accessible objective can help strengthen the confidence necessary to stay with a goal that calls for years of perseverance.

At an elevated level, such lucidity allows one to foresee how and when one's life will come to an end. Those who spend time with the dying say that when there is only one more month of life left, one thinks there are ten, the same thing for a week, a day, or an hour. However, premonition comes to the same result instantaneously.

sopakramaṃ nirupakramaṃ ca karma
tatsaṃyamādaparāntajñānamarṣṭiebhyo va
sopakramaṃ nirupakramaṃ ca karma
tat-saṃyamāt-aparānta-jñānam-ariṣṭebhyaḥ va

Sopakramam: with rapid evolution. *Nirupakramam:* with slow evolution. *Ca:* and. *Karma:* action. *Tat:* that. *Saṃyamāt:* through perfect mastery. *Aparānta:* final ending. *Jñānam:* knowledge. *Ariṣṭebhyaḥ:* portent. *Va:* or else by.

Perfect mastery of friendship and other qualities confers corresponding power.

Am I a solitary, even friendless person, or am I much sought after? Why?

How do others see me, and eventually, what do they reproach me with?

What quality should I develop?

What is the role of a positive mental attitude in teaching yoga? In therapy?

What is the connection between friendliness, contentedness (II.42), and the four positive mental attitudes (I.33)?

How can I prevent a positive attitude from becoming exaggerated optimism?

Why does Patañjali use the the word "friendship" in this aphorism?

This aphorism is based on one essential idea: in order to receive, we must first give.

Often the person who feels lonely, unloved, or disrespected is the one who finds it difficult to express friendly feelings or respect for others. By observing reproaches we would like to make to others, we should be able to discover qualities we need to develop ourselves. As children so rightly say: "Who says it, is it."

Sometimes, we might need a support for this discovery, whether verbal, conceptual, or visual. Looking at a picture of a being full of compassion for example, can favor the unfolding of that same quality in oneself with corresponding radiance. Charisma is at the origin of positive influence, of education, often even of healing, and quite obviously, of the flowing personality.

maitryādiṣu balāni
maitri-ādiṣu balāni

Maitri: friendship. *Ādiṣu:* etcetera. *Balāni:* the forces.

III.24

By perfect concentration on the elephant and other models, one gains their corresponding strengths.

What qualities do I lack, and what models can help me acquire them?

How can these models be of concrete use?

How can I prevent negative characteristics from arising as I concentrate on a model?

How can we prevent loss of identity when imitating a model?

Why is it necessary to use an actual model with physical characteristics?

This aphorism was written in a culture that had close contact with nature. In our age, what models would suit a town dweller living out of touch with nature?

In the preceding aphorism, Patañjali advised positive thought to obtain strength or moral qualities. In this aphorism, to develop physical qualities, he recommends long periods of concentration on a concrete model, such as an animal, that embodies those qualities. For example, the elephant is strong, the snake is supple, and so on. In this way, we become like the model. Such a phenomenon is related to imitation and its mode of action. Of course we never develop the exact physical qualities of the model, but we develop our maximum potential.

This course of action implies as much confidence as patience. The most important thing, therefore, is the choice of model.

baleṣu hastibalādīni
baleṣu hasti-balādīni

Baleṣu: on the forces. *Hasti:* elephant. *Bala:* forces. *Ādīni:* etcetera.

Joining the intelligence of the heart with the overflowing of the mind brings knowledge of the subtle or causal, the hidden or unusual, and the physically and psychologically remote.

Is it difficult for me to understand people of another generation, region, culture, or profession? What about those who are more subtle or sensitive than me? What should I do about it?

Is even the intelligence of the heart limited?

The intelligence of the heart is often the last level of the personality to awaken. What major difficulties must we overcome?

The mind enables us to understand tangible, visible, and accessible realities; its limitations quickly become apparent when we try to grasp subtleties, underlying causes, that which is hidden by our habits, and remote influences (from another generation, for example).

To attain realities out of its grasp, the mind must submerge itself in the intelligence of the heart. According to the Hindu tradition, the heart is where God dwells in human beings. And this aphorism signifies that a divine vision enlightens the mind.

As long as the ego is an obstacle in the personality, intellectual pride precludes the necessary abandonment. It is only in renouncing the qualities of the mind, however great they may be, that the intelligence of the heart may awaken. As Saint Exupry so justly says in *Le Petit Prince:* "You can only see with the heart."

pravṛttyālokanyāsātsūkṣmavyavahitaviprakṛṣṭajñānam
pravṛtti-āloka-nyāsāt-sūkṣma-vyavahita-viprakṛṣṭa-jñānam

Pravṛtti: manifestation. *Āloka:* shine, brilliance, constantly perceiving. *Nyāsāt:* through laying down, deposing. *Sūkṣma:* subtle, causal. *Vyavahita:* out of sight, habits. *Viprakṛṣṭa:* far away, far off, distant, remote physically or psychologically. *Jñānam:* knowledge.

III.26

Perfect concentration on the sun bestows knowledge of the universe.

How can I develop a spirit of synthesis?

What is the advantage of a spirit of synthesis in daily life? What is its disadvantage if pushed too far?

What is the relationship between this aphorism and the "Salute to the Sun" yoga posture practiced in many yoga schools?

In this aphorism and the next two, three objects of attention are proposed: the sun, the moon, and the polestar. Exploring the sun, the heavenly body at the center of the solar system, confers global knowledge of the system, that is, exploring the center of a system leads to general knowledge of the whole. In an organization, studying its director can more rapidly procure correct global knowledge of the whole setup. That is the spirit of synthesis.

In the Hindu tradition, the sun, *sūrya,* is one of the gods. He is surrounded by the *Veda.* Numerous prayers are addressed to him: the *gāyatrī* at dawn, *sāvitrī* at its zenith, *sarasvatī* at dusk. A Hindu prays to the sun to receive global knowledge of heaven and of its mythology—the seven worlds linked to the seven energy centers of the body (*cakras*). At the human level, the sun is in the heart. A *gāyatrī* is a prayer to bring the sun into the heart. This aphorism and the aphorism III.34 are therefore related. According to the Hindu tradition, the sun symbolizes man, and the moon, woman. By exploring the sun, we also explore the masculine aspect of a human being and the masculine pole of a couple. According to some traditions, the right side of the body is solar, the left side, lunar. Thereafter, exploring the sun consists in exploring the right side of the body. Lastly, in astrology, the sun's presence in a dwelling is another sector of inquiry.

bhuvanajñānam srūye saṃyamāt
bhuvana-jñānam srūye saṃyamāt

Bhuvana: of the world, the universe. *Jñānam:* knowledge. *Sūrye:* on the sun. *Saṃyamāt:* on account of perfect mastery.

Perfect concentration on the moon bestows knowledge of star patterns.

How can I develop my faculty of analysis? What are the advantages? If overdone, what disadvantages are likely?

How can exploring the mental state benefit someone actively engaged in life?

Is there a connection between this aphorism and I.40, which presented mastery of the infinitely small and the infinitely great?

In this aphorism, the object of research is the moon, the earth's satellite. Observing it leads to knowledge of the respective places occupied by the other elements in the solar system. It represents knowledge of the internal organization of the elements of a whole. This is the spirit of analysis, which complements the spirit of synthesis, represented by the sun. Using the example of the organization again, we are here observing the director's assistant, someone who takes charge of the actual organization.

In the Hindu tradition, the moon represents a goddess, Queen of the Night, related to the notion of sacred nectar (*amṛta*), the draught of immortality and sweetness. It also represents the psyche (*citta*), with its perpetual changes and explorations of the mind and its fluctuations.

The moon is the feminine pole of a couple and the left side of the body explored in the asymmetrical postures. Finally, in astrology, the moon is highly idiosyncratic. According to the *Taittirya Upaniṣad,* the moon proceeds from God's mental function, whereas the sun proceeds from God's eyes.

candre tārāvyūhajñānam
candre tārā-vyūha-jñānam

Candre: on, about the moon. *Tārā:* of the stars. *Vyūha:* disposal, arrangement, layout. *Jñānam:* knowledge.

III.28

Perfect concentration on the polestar bestows knowledge of the movement of the stars.

Do I have a stable point of reference with which to orient my evolution?

What qualities do I need to develop or find one?

What advantages can a stable life bring?

How can I prevent excessive immobility from degenerating into inertia?

Can having to be the fixed point in teaching relationships present disadvantages for personal evolution?

The third and last element of the whole, after sun and moon, the polestar is here proposed as a support for concentration.

Observing the sun affords global knowledge of a system, and the moon, understanding of a system's internal organization. Observing the polestar allows us to grasp the movements that animate the different elements within a system.

The polestar of the Little Bear constellation (Ursa Minor) is the fixed point that allows for observation of the heavenly bodies. It is also a guide for the observer's movement, for example navigating at sea. This aphorism leads to the search in society of a fixed point, remarkable for its stability: a wise person, a counselor, or some such person, who by his or her unwavering vision, permits observation of movements as a whole. In Indian tradition, permanence is ensured by the family's *guru,* whose advice backs up that of the father and the mother in the adolescent's education.

The polestar can represent the fixed point in any ethnic, cultural, social, professional, or family structure. The Indian marriage ceremony refers to the polestar, saying that marriage should be as firmly fixed as it is.

In every religion, dogma guarantees stability. In evolution through yoga, the student or disciple needs a point to fix on in order to discover and progressively diminish the fluctuations of the mind. Due to great personal stability, private life included, the teacher should be that point of reference.

dhruve tadgatijñānam
dhruve tad-gati-jñānam

Dhruve: the polestar, that which is fixed, invariable. *Tad:* that. *Gati:* of movement. *Jñānam:* knowledge.

Perfect concentration on the energy center of the navel affords knowledge of the body and its physiology.

How can concentrating on the navel:

- *help establish one's state of health?*
- *determine a specific yoga practice (postures or breathing rhythms)?*
- *link health and a balanced personality?*

How can we prevent deep and prolonged concentration on the navel area from becoming self-centeredness?

How can awareness of the navel area allow greater energy and better management of stress?

The intent of concentration on the navel is linked to the physical body and its energetic equivalents, for example, the energy centers (*cakra*) and other energetic levels in yoga and in Āyurveda. Other aphorisms refer to physical and energetic levels: the throat, III.30; the thorax, III.31; the top of the head, III.32; the heart, III.34; the throat on the energy level, III.39; and the center of the abdomen at the energy level, III.40.

Here, it is not a question of sitting down and gazing at one's navel, but of exploring this center of the physical body in all its aspects. According to the traditional medical systems of India and, in particular, according to the teacher T. Krishnamacharya, yoga and Āyurvedic specialist, the navel is the point of equilibrium, that is to say, the body's center of gravity. For a person of well-balanced build, the state of good health corresponds to an equilateral triangle formed by the navel and the two nipples.

Observing this zone imparts a great deal of information for diagnosis. Displacement of the navel:

- toward the bottom can indicate a blockage of the lower part of the trunk
- upward can indicate spasms in the region of the solar plexus
- to the left can indicate swollen liver or bile duct
- to the right can indicate swollen spleen

Manual exploration of the navel, the pains it can provoke, and the way they radiate also tell us about the state of health.

In fact, exploration of the navel gives information about the three humors: wind (*vāta*), bile (*pitta*), and phelgm (*kapha*), which are the expression of fluctuations in health.

According to yoga and to posture practice in particular, the navel is an important point. Posture directions, backward or forward, as well as breathing, modify the energy state of this zone.

Lastly, let us not forget the vital aspect of the navel:

- It is the link that ties the fetus to the mother.
- It is the energy center in certain martial arts.
- It is a symbol of equilibrium and of radiation of the personality in representations of the sacred.

nābhicakre kāyavyūhajñānam
nūbhi-cakre kāya-vyūha-jñānam

Nābhi: of the navel, the umbilicus. *Cakra:* bodily energy center, wheel, circle. *Kāya:* the body. *Vyūha:* disposition, arrangement. *Jñānam:* knowledge.

Perfect concentration on the throat frees one from hunger and thirst.

What has my relationship to food been until now? What could it be tomorrow; and what concrete approach can I take toward this objective?

What flavor attracts me most, and what is its influence on my health: sweet, salty, sour-acid, piquant, or bitter or astringent?

What should we do if attention to food becomes obsessive?

What consequences are likely, and how can one prevent these?

Is hunger an obstacle to my early morning yoga practice?

The observation here concerns the different channels that link the head to the trunk, in particular the esophagus (to the digestive tract). Hunger and thirst, the vital needs that link the individual to food and water can be felt in this area. Grafted onto this physical need for food and water is a psychological one: the need to change one's state of being after a period of activity. Thus, very often, we sit down to eat in order to change our psychological state.

Observing sensations in the throat, we choose hunger and the desire to satisfy it from the other sensations. The issue is not to suppress hunger and thirst, but to lessen dependence on them by choosing the moment and the quantity of nourishment ingested. Such an evolution often passes through four stages: ignorance, refusal to change, sticking to a diet that risks becoming an end in itself, and finally, good alimentary hygiene based on self-knowledge and judicious choices.

Such a process touches a deep-seated aspect that psychoanalysis calls "the oral stage." If it is true, as Estienne wrote (in 1593), that "the greedy dig their grave with their teeth," the theme of this aphorism is essential.

Such mastery favors health, suppleness and physical strength, mental clarity, and spiritual evolution.

kaṇṭhakūpe kṣutpipāsānivṛttiḥ
kaṇṭha-kūpe kṣut-pipāsā-nivṛttiḥ

Kaṇṭha: throat, neck. *Kūpe:* cavity, hole. *Kṣut:* hunger. *Pipāsā:* of thirst. *Nivṛttiḥ:* stoppage, ceasing.

III.31

Perfect concentration on the "tortoise channel" brings stability.

To develop confidence in myself, should I practice seated postures, with awareness on grounding?

How do stability, physical attitude, and voice relate to each other?

What qualities should accompany stability so that others flourish?

The tortoise channel is a subtle energy duct, assimilated with acupuncture meridians, that covers the front part of the trunk at the level of the sternum. This zone symbolizes courage in the face of adversity. Straightening the posture enables us to face aggression and difficulties. Emotion and fear, likely to show in the chest, give way to strength, energy, and stability through mental discipline or the practice of backward postures (opening postures).

In posture practice, the seated ones especially are likened in Hindu mythology to the tortoise, which supports the universe. The spinal column stands erect on this base. Focusing on the lower part of the body stabilizes a person. This is also true of the posture called "tortoise posture" with legs apart, face against the ground, and arms stretched out, passing under the knees.

The practice of breath control in a good seated position, and progressive mastery of the energy (*prāṇa*) located in the center of the thorax may also be related to this aphorism. For a Hindu, praying to the tortoise god, second incarnation of *Viṣṇu* and a symbol of stability, enables one to vanquish fear. Lastly, disapproval bends the back, while compliments strengthen the subtle energy in the tortoise channel and, at the same time, create stability.

kūrmanāḍyāṃ sthairyam
kūrma-nāḍyāṃ sthairyam

Kūrma: tortoise, the earth as a tortoise swimming in the waters, second reincarnation of Viṣṇu. *Nāḍyām:* channel. *Sthairyam:* stability, calm.

Perfect concentration on the spiritual light at the top of the head brings visions of realized beings.

What qualities can prepare me for this practice?

Can one venture into it alone, without regular advice from a guide?

What can regular contact with realized beings bring?

Does this aphorism imply a belief in the existence of invisible worlds?

What are the possible dangers of excessive endeavor in this direction?

According to yoga, intelligence and the sensory function come from a single source of light. During certain states of meditation, this light concentrates at the top of the head, in the area of one of the subtle energy centers, the *sahasrara cakra,* the lotus of a thousand petals (a thousand means infinite here).

This phenomenon enables us to enter relationships with certain beings endowed with clairvoyance. From that flows a better understanding of ourselves, our problems, and of others, as though these higher beings give us their help.

In short, concentrating on this light permits an approach of divine grace with the help of these mediators who are realized beings. The result may be likened to the action of divine grace.

Both the paranormal character of this aphorism and the extreme sensitivity of the energy center concerned call for a warning. This practice can be dangerous at the physical (circulatory) and psychological levels (stepping outside the body, etcetera), as well as to the spiritual one (illusion, ego).

mūrdhajyotiṣi siddhadarśanam
mūrdha-jyotiṣi siddha-darśanam

Mūrdha: the top of the head. *Jyotiṣi:* clarity, light as divine principle of life and source of intelligence. *Siddha:* a realized being, success, beatitude. *Darśanam:* vision, spiritual vision, point of view, doctrine.

III.33

Or else, through intuition, all is known.

Do people recognize me as someone having deep, correct, spontaneous insight—the fruit of natural intuition?

What elements in nature favor such faculties or weaken them, if necessary?

Does such a faculty correspond to a certain type of personality?

As we become more intuitive, how can we weigh which directions are favorable and which are not?

Does rational analysis of our intuitions answer the previous question?

After presenting a first method of apprehending life in a deeper, more subtle way in the preceding aphorism, Patañjali here suggests another alternative: direct grasp through intuition.

Whereas the first method entails a certain procedure, this one is spontaneous, springing from the heart. Such an experience is possible only if a person is established in the yoga state, also called the fourth state (*turya*). The other three states are wakefulness, sleep, and dreaming.

The grasp of realities that then occurs leaves all sensory perception behind and allows us to grasp practically everything. The intuitive knowledge that bubbles up is original, new, and unforgettable.

prātibhādvā sarvam
prātibhāt-vā sarvam

Prātibhāt: through, by intuition or premonition. *Vā:* or else by. *Sarvam:* all.

Perfect concentration on the heart reveals the contents of the mind.

What qualities can benefit my inquiry into the heart?

Must the heart be sufficiently pure before taking such a step?

Is great affective sensitivity an advantage or a handicap in such an investigation?

Does revealing the contents of thought through observing the heart happen only after thoughts slow down or even stop?

Is there a connection between this aphorism and devotion to God (varapraidhna, I.23)?

Why is exploration of the heart one of the last stages we can attain?

The Sanskrit word translated as "heart" (*hṛdayam*) does not really correspond to the heart muscle. It refers to a particularly sensitive area located at the midline and the base of the thorax. According to Āyurvedic medicine this area is related to:

- breathing and the ingestion of food (*prāṇa*)
- circulation of liquids and energy in the body (*vyāna*)
- memory and other mental functions (*sādhaka*)
- strength of the limbs (*avalambaka*)
- functioning of the sense organs (*tarpaka*)

Furthermore, according to the *Chāndogya-upaniṣad,* Chapter 8, the heart is where one perceives space (*ākāśa*); this *ākāśa* is the city of Brahman, or God, and desires. It is also said that the inner being (*ātman*) is in the heart. The sun, whose every ray speeds in the direction of each of the worlds, resides in the heart. During deep, dreamless sleep, each human being returns to the "dwelling of the heart" and is bathed in this divine, solar light. According to yoga, this heart corresponds to the fourth *cakra, ānahata,* which is dark red and which one may meditate on using the *yaṃ mantra.*

This heart is the center of the emotions and sentiments and also the starting point of life and regeneration. This links it closely to conscious thought. We could present the mind as the actor who plays what the heart writes. Henceforth, observing the heart region in detail allows us to grasp the origin of thoughts after, during, or even, someday, in anticipation of an event.

That this aphorism is not presented until the third chapter implies that a certain well-being is required to realize this experience (*sukha*). If the heart is full of anguish (*duḥkha*), we must undertake numerous intermediary practices or stages before undertaking this endeavor.

For a believer, this inquiry into the heart is one into God and corresponds to the prayer of the heart.

hṛdaye cittasaṃvit
hṛdaye citta-saṃvit

Hṛdaye: of the heart (also seat of the emotions). *Citta:* of the psyche, mind, intelligence, thought, sentiment, emotion. *Saṃvit:* complete knowledge, understanding.

The spiritual entity is independent of pacified consciousness. Confusing them only brings a reflection of the spiritual entity. Perfect concentration on their difference brings recognition of the spiritual entity.

Do my successes and failures totally determine my choices in existence?

How can I detach from the results of my actions?

What brings us closer to this experience:

- *self-reflection?*
- *psychological work, one on one or in a group?*
- *examining my conscience?*
- *a succession of setbacks in life?*
- *a spiritual practice?*

How can we distinguish authentic discovery of the self from egocentrism?

If we accept two levels of individual being—spiritual and material, including the psyche and thought—how is each level reflected in the words "I" and "myself" used in the following expressions:

- *I am interested in myself?*
- *I think of myself?*
- *I observe myself?*

What are the advantages and disadvantages of perpetually questioning oneself?

What are the connections between this aphorism, action yoga, (karma yoga), and the yoga of knowledge (jñāna-yoga)?

Is there a link between this experience and vairāgya (I.12)?

This aphorism describes a radical change of objectives within the personality.

A human being who is not lucid, or a believer who does not perceive spiritual presence within, follows a host of outer objectives. His or her choices are determined by experiences of pleasure and suffering.

When one attains the level described here, however, a continual sense of presence within reveals a single objective, however the intent difffers: progressive discovery of the self or, for the believer, of the spiritual entity.

Whether the result of our actions is successful or not, only one thing counts: What have I learned?"

The way proposed here is none other than that famous "Know thyself and thou shalt know the universe and the gods," attributed to Socrates.

As long as pleasure is directed toward the outer world, such an endeavor is impossible. This stage, so difficult to cross, corresponds to a total reversal of objectives. It takes a very long time.

sattvapuruṣayoḥ atyantāsaṅkīrṇayoḥ pratyayāviśeṣo bhogaḥ
parārthatvātsvārthasaṁyamātpuruṣajñānam.
sattva-puruṣayoḥ atyantā-asaṅkīrṇayoḥ pratyaya-aviśeṣaḥ-bhogaḥ
parārthatvāt-svārtha-saṁyamāt-puruṣa-jñānam

Sattva: the mental in an understanding state, of transparency, clarity, one of the three constituent qualities of nature (I.16). *Puruṣayoḥ:* of the spiritual principle (inherent to everyone). *Atyantā*: beyond all limits, extremely. *Asaṅkīrṇayoḥ:* unmixed, distinct. *Pratyaya:* experience (at the level of consciousness), contents of the mind. *Aviśeṣaḥ:* indistinct (indistinct), undifferentiated. *Bhogaḥ:* enjoyment on the level of sentiment, experience as lived. *Parārthatvāt:* because of another aim. *Svārtha:* interest in the higher Being. *Saṁyamāt:* because of perfect concentration. *Puruṣa:* of the spiritual principle. *Jñānam:* knowledge.

It is then that the faculties of premonition, clairaudience, subtle touch, clairvoyance, refined taste, and sensitive sense of smell appear.

What attitude should I take toward my experience of these powers?

How can I avoid seeking these faculties?

Are such phenomena inevitable once we become conscious of the inner being?

What personality traits can interfere with this kind of perception (II.3)?

In daily life, the sense organs take in the surroundings more or less accurately. The intent to direct the sense organs toward objects is necessary for perception, but limits it. Although the desire to perceive is indispensable, it gets in the way by coloring perception and lessening objectivity. It can hamper any intuitive perception of what is out of range for the sense organs.

When one no longer seeks external results, and the intent of perception becomes self-discovery, the perceiving entity in the depths of oneself begins to perceive objects out of normal range of the sense organs. Seeking to perceive while detached from exterior results favors clairvoyance. The order in which the six powers are presented here follows the order of the *āṃkhya,* from the subtlest to the grossest: premonition, hearing, touch, sight, taste, and smell, corresponding to the basic elements: ether, air, fire, water, and earth.

tataḥ prātibhaśrāvaṇavedanādarśāsvādavārtā jāyante
tataḥ prātibha-śrāvaṇa-vedana-ādarśa-āsvāda-vārtā jāyante

Tata: then, following then, afterward. *Prātibha:* intuition, premonition, foreknowledge. *Śrāvaṇa:* clairaudience. *Vedana:* subtle touch. dara: clairvoyance. *Āsvāda:* refined taste. *Vārtāḥ:* subtle sense of smell. *Jāyante:* are produced, appear.

III.37

These faculties are obstacles in contemplation, but powers in active life.

If such faculties appear in me, should I:

- *ignore them or push them aside?*
- *develop them and use them to benefit others?*
- *keep a noncomittal and discreet attitude?*

How can we prevent them inflaming old, negative impulses, such as fear, repulsion, attachment, and ego?

Is renunciation one way to deal with this?

This aphorism is the first to warn against negative effects that accompany these powers. All acquisition of power, faculties, or responsibilities in one's life carries with it the risks of attachment and loss of liberty. We never know beforehand how someone will respond to new powers and responsibilities.

Acquiring extraordinary faculties gives rise to an outburst of mental activity that produces creative action. Such powers are then a great help. However, the sudden, unforeseeable appearance of extrasensory perception, and flashes of the future, images, scenes, and music, can inflame negative impulses (*kleśa,* II.3). One may experience fears when faced with certain frightening scenes, excessive repulsion or attachment when faced with certain visions, or a feeling of pride.

Thereafter, it is better not to seek these powers. Too much playing hooky, whatever the pleasure, makes the road longer, and the goal much further off. This aphorism applies not only to the extrasensory powers presented here, but to the powers in this chapter as a whole.

te samādhāvupasargā vyutthāne siddhayaḥ
te samādhau-upasargāḥ vyutthāne siddhayaḥ

Te: these latter. *Samādhau:* in contemplation. *Upasargāḥ:* of obstacles, of unhappiness. *Vyutthāne:* in activity. *Siddhayaḥ:* of powers, of accomplishments, of realizations.

Letting go of the structure of personality and refining perception of movement awakens the faculty of influencing another's mind and body.

Do I have natural authority, that is, do I strongly influence others?

Does my family or professional situation require me to influence others positively?

If need be, how can I develop my influence?

What keeps me from accepting my personality and my social, religious, and family origins?

How can I overcome these obstacles?

What personal erroneous leanings (II.3) might stem from using these powers or even lead to using them inappropriately?

How do I overcome these dangers?

To what extent does teaching yoga imply such a faculty?

The beginning of Chapter IV of the *Yoga Sūtras* deals with the role of one's influence over others in constructing and evolving the personality. Patañjali here sets out conditions that allow such influence: the possibility of inhabiting another's body with one's mind.

Used in a negative way, this faculty enables one to manipulate another like a puppet, unknown to that person. Used in a positive manner, however, it is indispensable in helping others out of personal difficulties and to rebuild their lives.

Personality takes its shape gradually under many influences, those of parents notably. Accepting our character and making peace with the influences that shaped it (for example, society, religion, parents, or past actions) constitute the first condition of liberty that will enable us to influence another.

The second condition is refining our perceptions until, gradually, we can perceive previously invisible movements that give life to the physical body. Such a process may be summed up in four stages.

1. letting go of conditioning
2. subtly grasping another's behavior
3. adapting to the other's behavior
4. changing the other's behavior by changing one's own

As long as one is self-conflicted, there is no place for others and one has no influence over them.

bandhakāraṇaśaithilyātpracārasaṃvedanācca
cittasya paraśarīrveśaḥ
bandha-kāraṇa-śaithilyāt-pracāra-saṃvedanāt-ca
cittasya para-śarīra-āveśaḥ

Bandha: focusing, binding, attaching. *Kāraṇa:* cause, origin. *Śaithilyāt:* because of relaxing, relaxing, pacification. *Pracāra:* movement. *Saṃvedanāt:* because of subtle perception. *Ca:* and. *Cittasya:* of the psyche, of the mind, intelligence, thought, sentiment, emotion. *Para:* other. *Śarīra:* body. *Āveśaḥ:* entry, entrance, entering, penetration, taking possession of.

With perfect mastery of rising vital energy, one rises above water, mud, and thorns.

Do my difficulties seem light to me?

Does my voice ring out clearly in public when necessary, or do I often have throat problems?

What is the role of chanting and the voice in my practice, in light of this aphorism?

What kind of relationship links udāna with spiritual elevation?

Yogis distinguish several kinds of energy, including the rising vital energy (*udāna*) at the level of the throat. This is the energy of spirtual elevation and brings speech and the skill, or faculty, of avoiding and overcoming obstacles. It is also, according to Hindu tradition, the energy that leaves the body through the top of the head at the moment of death.

Speech may be clear, or it may be thick with emotion, either because of excessive saliva (water), mucus (mud), or sudden irritation (thorns). The feeling of lightness and ease, as this energy rises, enables us to avoid accidents due to water, mud, and thorns, both in the real sense and in the figurative sense (the confusion of others or certain traits for which we are the target).

Mastery of *udāna* thus permits good elocution, the knack of avoiding certain obstacles and, at the limit, influence over one's death.

udānajayjājalapaṅkakaṇṭakādiṣvasaṅga utkrāntiśca
udāna-jayāt-jala-paṅka-kaṇṭaka-ādiṣu-asaṅgaḥ utkrāntiḥ-ca

Udāna: one of the five breaths,* rising vital energy. *Jayāt:* by mastery of. *Jala:* water. *Paṅka:* mud. *Kaṇṭaka:* thorns. *Ādiṣu:* etc., and soon. *Asaṅgaḥ:* without contact. *Utkrānthi:* ascension. *Ca:* and.

*The five breaths are *prāṇa,* vital energy in all its forms, and its four principal manifestations; *apāna* (elimination), *samāna* (assimilation and equilibrium), *udāna* (elevation), *vyāna* (diffusion), *Śiva-Saṃhitā* (III.2 to III.7) and *Gheraṇḍa-saṃhitā* (V.60, V.61, V.62).

III.40

Perfect mastery of the vital energy of assimilation and equilibrium brings radiance.

How can developing and purifying the vital energy in the abdomen increase my radiance?

What are the risks of focusing too much energy on the two extremes of the trunk (head and genitals)?

Are there obstacles to recentering at the area of the navel?

What methods to refocus my energy best suit me: practice of prāṇāyāma; careful diet, or meditation on the navel area?

What are the signs that energies are refocusing?

Mastering the vital energy of assimilation and equilibrium (*samāna*) involves successful *prāṇāyāma* practice with suspension of breath and *bandhas* to generate heat in the navel area. *Samāna* is situated in the region of the navel (III.34) and is the meeting point of the two breaths observed during *prāṇāyāma.*

Prāṇāyāma elevates *apāna,* the breath of elimination and brings down *prāṇa,* vital energy (*Haṭha yoga pradīpikā* II.47), or sacrificing one of these breaths on the altar of the navel (*Bhagavad Gītā,* IV.29). Digestion takes place in this area through the action of the digestive juices (*jvalanam* in Sanskrit, meaning radiant heat). Refocusing this energy increases the temperature of the body center, favors elimination, and becomes radiant heat. One may refer back to the three aphorisms of this text that address *prāṇāyāma*—II.49, II.50, and II.51.

Meditation on the fire element, a red triangle shape between the navel and the heart, with the essential sound (*bīja mantra*) *RAṂ,* can be a means of attaining mastery of *samāna* (*Mantramahodadhī,* I.13 to I.18).

samānajayājjvalanam
samāna-jayāt-jvalanam

Samāna: one of the five breaths, vital energy of assimilation and equilibrium (see notes in the preceding aphorism). *Jayāt:* through conquest, victory. *Jvalanam:* radiance.

Perfect mastery of the relationship between the ear and space brings extraordinary hearing.

Do I have a quick ear or am I hard of hearing?

How can I improve my hearing:

- *by focusing on the relationship between the ear and space?*
- *by paying more attention to the person I am speaking with?*
- *with exercises in inner listening?*
- *with methods that use sound or chanting?*

How does hearing relate to age and to family surroundings?

Am I interested in hearing, touching, seeing everything, and so on?

Is there a connection between aphorisms I.15 (heard objects), III.7 (the internal quality of the last three limbs), and this one?

Extraordinary hearing is not the understanding of information received, but the perfect reception of sounds. In everyday life, we sometimes hear without hearing, catching only part of what is said. Refusing to listen to another can even lead to partial deafness, with the attention remaining stuck on an inner discourse or on other exterior sounds.

This faculty consists in hearing totally and exactly what is said. It is influenced by the practice of music, chanting, and so on. This refinement of perception applies also to the other senses: touch, taste, sight, and smell, and also to actions (speech, grip, locomotion, excretion, and enjoyment).

If attention to the relationship between the space around sounds and the reception of sound by the ear refines acuteness of hearing, then, according to T. Krishnamacharya, hearing is only possible through power—the energy of the inner spiritual entity.

śrotrākāśyoḥ saṃbandhasaṃyamāddivyaṃ śrotram
śrotra-ākāśyoḥ saṃbandha-saṃyamāt-divyaṃ śrotram

Śrotra: the ear, hearing. *Ākāśayo:* ether, spaceone of the five elements that constitute the universe. *Saṃbandha:* of relationship. *Saṃyamāt:* from perfect mastery. *Divyam*: divine. *Śrotram:* hearing (*ātman*).

III.42

Mastering the relationship between the body and ether, then meditating on the lightness of cotton, brings displacement in space.

Am I perfectly at ease when I am traveling or adapting to a fresh environment?

Can I develop this quality in a way that doesn't destroy an already uprooted personality?

Is this way of proceeding dangerous for certain people?

How can I avoid losing my sense of reality when I experience this power?

What practices should accompany the appearance of this faculty?

Our physical and mental experiences of weight are different: "I feel so heavy," or "I am lighthearted." When enclosed in the seed, cotton is heavy, but the cotton ball, once teased out, flies away at the slightest puff of wind. Meditating on such an image favors the growth of a feeling of lightness.

Such a state, linked to awareness of the relationship between the body and space (ether), allows the feeling that the body is dissolving in a given place, and reconstituting in another. Any element that favors the feeling of lightness may be used: awareness of the void, exercises of expanding consciousness, and so on.

The feeling of heaviness inhibits; the feeling of lightness confers great freedom to travel, move about, and make the changes and transformations that are indispensable to life. One's constitution (*prakṛti*) influences this faculty. A preponderance of wind (*vāta*) facilitates the feeling of lightness, whereas phlegm (*kapha*) can be a handicap (see commentary, I.22).

kāyākāśayoḥ saṃbandhasaṃyamāllaghutūlasamāpatteś cākāśagamanam
kāyā-kāśayoḥ saṃbandha-saṃyamāt-laghu-tūla-samāpatteḥ ca-ākāśa-gamanam

Kāya: body. *Ākāśayoḥ:* ether, space. *Sabandha:* on, about relationship. *Saṃyamāt:* because of perfect mastery. *Laghu:* light, quick. *Tūla:* cotton. *Samāpatteḥ:* meditation. *Ca:* and. *Ākāśa:* ether, space. *Gamanam:* moving about.

When outside things no longer condition mental activity, the veil over the light of understanding is rent asunder and a state of liberation appears.

What can I do if fear, aggression, attachment, or the ego condition my thoughts, words, and actions?

What does this expression imply: Give yourself a good conscience in order to act?

What part of an action is due to motives and what part to justification after the event?

How does this aphorism relate to confusion and lucidity, or to inhibition and overactivity?

Is there a contradiction between compassion and emotional restraint in service to others?

Is there a connection between this aphorism and nonattachment (I.16)?

A clear and immediate vision of reality calls for a mode of mental functioning different from the usual one. When we receive a piece of information, we usually speculate—an action steeped in affectivity. Our thoughts and actions are external in two ways: they concern what is outside the body; and although they occur inside the body, they lie outside the spiritual entity. Every habitual action and thought is the result of interaction between these two "outsides."

The unconditioned mind receives information without being shaped by anything exterior, and action is independent of a person's erroneous leanings (*kleśa,* II.3). At this exceptional level of awareness things take place thus: I see, I know I should be able to act, and I act on another's account and at his or her request. Being within another dimension, one no longer needs the gratification of one's acts. Action based on self-interest vanishes.

bahirakalpitā vṛttirmahāvidehā tataḥ prakāśāvaraṇakṣayaḥ
bahiḥ-akalpitā vṛttiḥ-mahāvidehā tataḥ prakāśa-āvaraṇa-kṣayaḥ

Bahiḥ: outside. *Akalpitā:* unconceived, not conceived. *Vṛttiḥ:* fluctuations of the mind. *Mahāvidehā:* the state where one is free from the body. *Tataḥ:* then, thereafter. *Prakāśa:* light. *Āvaraṇa:* veil. *Kṣayaḥ:* destruction.

III.44

Mastering the material—the real form, the causal structure, concrete possibilities, and value based on the goal—brings mastery of the five elements.

Are my physique and my health balanced?

What improvements are possible and what can I hope for?

How can I make these happen?

To what extent can we foresee which foods or surroundings will affect us?

Does this aphorism help us reduce only self-induced suffering?

How can we experiment, yet stay detached?

Is there a connection between this aphorism and aphorisms III.13 (changing realites) and III.43 (unconditioned mind)?

According to yoga, nature (including our bodies) is made up of five primary elements:

- Ether holds the principle of space, or what is void or hollow.
- Air holds the principle of gas and movement.
- Fire holds the principle of heat and metabolism.
- Water holds the principle of what is liquid and fluid.
- Earth holds the principle of what is solid and dense.

The density of these five primary elements varies for each organ in the body. When their proportion corresponds to the given organ, they are balanced, and we are healthy. States of imbalance or illness may stem from three sources: from nature, from others, or from oneself (see the commentary in II.15). This aphorism shows us how to prevent disorders that stem from ourselves—mistakes we make through activities, leisure pursuits, food, and so on.

Take the Water element, or body fluids, for example: When there is too little (for example, dry lacrimal glands) or too much (for example, congested lymphatic system) severe illness can occur. Another example is imbalance of Earth, which maintains volume and body weight: too much may lead to obesity, too little to anorexia.

The five primary elements dance constantly with one another to maintain balance. The means proposed in this aphorism helps us to develop our awareness through direct experimentation. For example, using Water:

- What is its crude nature (*sthūla*)?
- What are its properties? What happens if we drink more or less (*svarūpa*)?

- What is the significance of water on the causal level? Why do we want to drink or not? How does the liquid act at all body levels (*sūkṣma*)?
- How does the proportion of body fluids affect the other four elements? How do the elements regulate and balance each other?
- How does our state of mind (inertia, activity, or equilibrium) affect the way liquids act in the body? Can too much water lead to heaviness or inertia (*anvaya*)?
- With regard to liberation, how important is it to enjoy the experience? What is the motive (*arthavattva,* II.18)? What if one backs away?

This aphorism presents the way to manage our health by paying attention to the basic elements that make up the body. Patañjali proposes daily experimentation, including analyzing our motives.

Āyurvedic medicine has explored the depths of this domain, drawing a parallel between a flavor, for example, and its action on the five primary elements (see the following table and the commentary in aphorism I.22).

sthūlasvarūpasūkṣmānvayārthavattvasaṃyamādbhūtajayaḥ
sthūla-svarūpa-sūkṣmā-ānvayā-arthavattva-saṃyamāt-bhūtaj-ayaḥ

Sthūla: coarse, unrefined, gross, material. *Svarūpa:* real shape, form, physical property. *Sūkṣma:* subtle structure, build, causal level. *Anvaya*: interpenetration, interplay, concrete, real possibility. *Arthavattva:* the value, based on the aim. *Saṃyamāt:* because, on account of perfect mastery. *Bhūta:* primary element. *Jayaḥ:* mastery, correct management.

Flavors and Their Actions on the Five Primary Elements

FLAVORS	QUALITIES	EMOTIONS	DOMINANT ELEMENTS	EQUILIBRIUM	EXCESS
sweet	heavy, damp, fresh	love, attachment	earth-water	vāta-pitta	kapha
salty	burning, damp, heavy	covetousness	water-fire	vāta	pitta-kapha
sour-acid	heavy, damp, burning	envy	earth-fire	vāta	pitta-kapha
piquant	hot, light, dry	repulsion, hate	air-fire	kapha	pitta-vāta
bitter	fresh, light, dry	rancor	air-ether	kapha-pitta	vāta
astringent	fresh, light, dry	fear	earth-air	pitta-kapha	vāta

Perfect mastery of the five elements brings mastery of physical form, physical vigor, and freedom from physical constraint.

Is my body an obstacle or an instrument that allows me to blossom?

What concrete actions can help me tune this instrument?

Is this physical blossoming embarrassing or does it encourage others?

How can I use this physical vigor in service to others?

How can I prevent this mastery from boosting my ego and making me overly interested in my own body?

Does this aphorism mean that a yogi is never ill?

How do I avoid getting carried away with dreams and fantasies about these powers?

Can a yoga adept interrupt a regular practice for several days and still find a glimmer of understanding of this aphorism?

What is the connection between this aphorism and III.42 (displacement in space)?

This aphorism shows us what mastery of the five elements brings. It emphasizes that the faculties acquired should be applied first to one's own body. In his commentary, Vyāsa lists eight such powers:

1. *Aṇimā:* miniaturization, or the faculty of reducing body volume
2. *Laghimā:* lightness, or the possibility of reducing weight
3. *Mahimā:* expansion, or the faculty of growth
4. *Prāpti:* vastness, or the possibility of reaching all
5. *Prākāmya:* irresistible willpower that enables one to overcome obstacles
6. *Vaśītva:* mastery over the body's constituent elements and their source
7. *Īśittva:* control of the materialization or dematerialization of elements
8. *Yatrakāmāvaśāyitva:* the possibility of determining the nature of elements, that is, transmuting one into another

This aphorism makes it quite clear that physical blossoming is marked by the absence of chemical, physical and other laws that govern our bodies. From then on, the faculties listed above may be more or less extraordinary, but they themselves remain subject to these laws. It is through discovery, knowledge, and good management of these laws, that these eight extraordinary powers appear.

What remains, however, is that such a blossoming confers a liberty of thought and action in life that is far superior to anything before, because the body has become a perfectly attuned and obedient instrument. He (or she) is in great shape, as the popular expression so aptly puts it.

tato'ṇimādiprādurbhāvaḥ kāyasaṃpattaddharmānabhighātaśca
tataḥ-aiṇma-ādi-prādurbhāvaḥ kāya-saṃpat-tad-dharma-anabhighātaḥ-ca

Tataḥ: then, following that. *Aṇima:* miniaturization. *Ādi:* etc. and so on. *Prādurbhāvaḥ:* manifestation. *Kāya:* body, physical form. *Saṃpat:* blooming plenitude. *Tad:* that (referring to the body). *Dharma:* order, law, foundation, structure. *Anabhighātaḥ:* indestructibility. *Ca:* and.

Physical plenitude consists in physical beauty, charm, strength, and being as solid as a diamond.

Does my way of doing yoga produce at least partial results? If not, what is at fault?

How can I prevent an overly materialistic bent toward this physical and personal blooming?

How can I attain a happy medium and stick to it with regard to each of these qualities?

How can I transcend this power?

The list of different qualities (III.45) that appear with physical blossoming emphasizes the concrete character of this power. These qualities should, therefore, become physically evident for the yoga adept.

It goes without saying that if we start yoga during adolescence, the results develop rapidly and more obviously than with an older beginner. However, even an older person can slow, or stop, or even provisionally reverse the physical aging of certain organs.

This aphorism seems to have been written in reply to the future demands of many westerners. In effect, yoga is often presented in the West as a way aiming at beauty, strength, and physical stamina.

rūpalāvaṇyabalavajrasaṃhananatvāni kāyasapat
rūpa-lāvaṇya-bala-vajra-saṃhananatvāni kāya-saṃpat

Rāpa: form, shape, beauty. *Lāvaṇya:* attraction, attractiveness, charm. *Bala:* power, strength. *Vajra:* diamond, thunderbolt. *Saṃhananatvāni:* firmness, solidity, endurance. *Kāya:* body, physical appearance. *Saṃpat:* blossoming, fullness, plenitude.

III.47

Perfect mastery of perception, of the perceived object, of the perceiving entity, of the reference in oneself, and of the intent, brings mastery of the organs of perception, action, and thought.

What can I learn from the following questions:

- *What do I see?*
- *What do I understand?*
- *Am I conscious of understanding?*
- *Am I aware of the particular features in me that allow understanding?*
- *What is my intent?*

What erroneous tendencies of the personality (II.3) get in the way of such mastery?

How important is the choice of objects before setting off on the conquest of the sense organs?

Is it better to choose objects that correspond to one's strong points (seen objects for a visual temperament) or one's weak points (sounds for a visual temperament)?

Can thinking about the organs of perception, action, thought, and their corresponding elements (according to the Sāṃkhya) be useful?

How important is control of the organs of perception, action, and thought in human relations, and in particular, in teaching yoga?

Is there a connection between this aphorism and the fifth limb of yoga—withdrawal from the sense organs (pratyāhāra, II.54)?

The extraordinary power presented in this aphorism concerns the immense frontier between an individual and his or her surroundings, that is, the sense organs.

Yoga adopts the sense organs of the *Sāṃkhya* system in their entirety. This system presents them in correspondence with the primary elements and the sensitive qualities. The following classification thus reveals eleven sense organs: five of perception, five of action, and a managing organ—the thought function.

Classification of Eleven Sense Organs

Sensory Faculties	Organs	Faculties of Action	Organs	Qualities	Primary Sensible Elements
hearing	ears	speech, voice	phonatory apparatus	sonorous	ether, space
touch	skin	grip	hand	tangible	air, movement
sight	eyes	locomotion	feet	visible	fire-heat, light
taste	tongue, palate	excretion	anus	sapid	water, liquid
smell	nose	enjoyment	sex	olfactory	earth, matter
thought reflex					

Take the example of reading: Sight permits us to receive a message made up of calligraphic signs (ink, paper) (*grahaṇa*).

On the second level, this message gives rise to understanding, or identification (*svarūpa*).

A possible third level is awareness of what one understands: for example, "I see, I understand." Such understanding is more or less clear depending on how detached one is with regard to what has just been read (*asmitā*).

At the fourth level we discover that we take in information only because it awakens references in us: knowledge of the written language. The object, the mental, and the "perceiving entity" (*anvaya*) interact with each other.

The fifth and last level is the reason why—the intent—to be translated in terms of enjoyment or of liberation: To what extent am I completely absorbed by the message read? To what extent am I detached or fully conscious of my free will? In brief, what is the final outcome (*arthavattva*)?

Perfect mastery of the sense organs is very difficult to achieve and maintain as long as it remains linked to the three constituent qualities of nature (*guṇas*) and their fluctuations. However, it is the doorway to the stages of inner yoga—those of meditation.

grahaṇasvarūpasmitānvayārthavattvasaṃyamād-
indriyajàyaḥ
grahaṇa-svarūpa-asmitā-anvaya-arthavattva-saṃyamāt-
indriya-jaya˙

Grahaṇa: instrument of perception, sensory perception. *Svarūpa:* real nature. *Asmitā:* individual consciousness. *Anvaya:* relation. *Arthavattva:* meaning, aim. *Saṃyamāt:* through, by perfect mastery of concentration. *Indriya:* organs of perception, action, or thought. *Jayaḥ:* victory, conquest.

Then, instantaneous thought, perception independent of the sense organs, and perfect mastery of origins appear.

Do others see me as spontaneous, free and conscious of where my emotions, speech, and actions come from?

Does attaining instantaneous thought mean I will no longer waste my time seeking solutions to problems?

How can the sense organs enslave us?

Does independence from the sense organs mean that I will no longer need them (extrasensory perception) or that they are at our command?

What is the role of freedom in teaching yoga?

It often happens that one thinks over a problem in the evening and its solution comes to mind on waking. We have two types of mental functioning, a progressive one and an instantaneous one. Permanent, instantaneous thought is the first result presented here.

Perception independent of the sense organs means that the body and the sense organs no longer present obstacles to perception and action, but are obedient and used with pertinence. Don't some handicapped people do better than a great many in sound health?

Mastery of origins, the last result, enables us, through knowledge of the primary cause of events, to manage them better. Surely it is much easier to overcome a fire when it first breaks out than several hours later, or else to bend a sapling rather than a hundred-year-old oak. Seizing the primary cause confers liberty of action.

Sometimes people say that yoga leads to a mastery that kills spontaneity. This aphorism proves the contrary. If, at first, it seems to emphasize attention and diminish spontaneity, it afterwards becomes correct and total once more.

tato manojavitvaṃ vikaraṇabhāvaḥ pradhānajayaśca
tataḥ manaḥ-javitvaṃ vikaraṇa-bhāvaḥ pradhāna-jayaḥ-ca

Tataḥ: then, thereafter. *Manaḥ:* thought. *Javitvam:* instantaneousness. *Vikaraṇa:* independence of the sense organs. *Bhāvaḥ:* the state. *Pradhāna:* the primary cause. *Jayaḥ*: victory. *Ca:* and.

III.49

Complete revelation of the difference between the perceiving entity and the mind at peace brings omniscience and omnipotence.

How can I remain detached from my growing competence?

Why do we have to give up something of ourselves in order to receive something else? Who gives up? And from whom do we receive?

What preliminary conditions encourage us to be positive in our questioning?

What are the dangers of omniscience and omnipotence?

Through yoga we gradually attain peaceful mind and lucidity about ourselves and others. The personality stabilizes. At a high level, the individual keeps this inner stability whatever the surrounding disturbances may be. Patañjali uses the word *sattva,* equilibrium, for this mental function, for it remains in this state.

This high level presents one disadvantage, the risk of thinking we need go no further. By remaining aware of this obstacle, by going beyond the difference between the field of consciousness at peace and Absolute Consciousness, we merge with the omniscience and omnipotence that stems from that Absolute.

Any trace of ego is a screen. The road to this distinction is non-stop questioning of what is and is not my true nature: "Who am I?" If I reply "I am so and so," then who is speaking? No matter how clear-sighted and pacified, the mental remains the mental.

Such states of omniscience and omnipotence are not yet permanent, but they become so, as described in the aphorisms that follow.

sattvapuruṣānyatākhyātimātrasya sarvabhāvādhiṣṭhātṛtvaṃ sarvajñātṛtvaṃ ca
sattva-puruṣa-anyatā-khyāti-mātrasya sarva-bhāva - adhiṣṭhāttvaṃ sarvajñātṛtvaṃ ca

Sattva: state of mental peace. *Puruṣa:* Spiritual Entity. *Anyatā:* fundamental difference. *Khyāti:* complete recognition. *Mātrasya:* only, alone. *Sarvabhāva:* complete state of. *Adhiṣṭhātṛtvam:* supremacy. *Sarvajttvam:* omniscience. *Ca:* and.

Spiritual liberation comes when we renounce even omniscience and omnipotence, and when the origin of personal causes of suffering is destroyed.

What can I do to prevent myself, after a success, from thinking I've made it?

What is the role of renunciation in spiritual evolution?

What does the popular expression, "the more you know, the less you say," mean to me?

Is there a link between omniscience and omnipotence?

How can I avoid fearing my powers or desiring them?

The impurities or blemishes (*doṣas*) in question here are the five personal causes of suffering (*kleśas*) listed in the beginning of Chapter II: misconception, ego, attachment, aversion, and fear.

It is natural that with the appearance of omniscience and omnipotence we can see the reappearance of such afflictions as pride in having these powers, attachment to them, aversion to those in whom we see disastrous attitudes, or even fear of premonitions of dramatic events.

If omniscience and omnipotence bring the slightest trace of ego in their wake, the least pleasure or passion, as well as aversion or fear, we quickly lose our head and stumble. We must be extremely careful to get over this last obstacle and realize spiritual liberation.

tadvairāgyādapi doṣabījakṣaye kaivalyam
tad-vairāgyād-api doṣa-bīja-kṣaye kaivalyam

Tad: that (omnipotence and omniscience). *Vairāgyāt:* because of nonattachment. *Api:* the same, as well. *Doṣa:* blemish, stain. *Bīja:* root, seed. *Kṣaye:* destruction. *Kaivalyam:* spiritual liberation.

III.51

When higher creatures invite you, do not give way to wonderment on meeting them, but keep a detached viewpoint when faced with their allure.

Am I often invited by the great ones of this world (or of the next)?

How can I decide which invitations to accept?

What should my attitude be toward accepting or refusing the invitation?

What sort of personal interests are likely to induce us to accept such invitations?

What sort of discipline is necessary to ignore them?

Does refusing honors mean that one has gotten over this pitfall?

The flowering of the qualities described in the preceding aphorism necessarily entail numerous invitations from the great ones of the world who wish to be honored by our presence. In a more mystical context, apparitions and visions can occur.

The danger is not in accepting these invitations or not, but in how we view the time. However, accepting such invitations can often influence or weaken the state of withdrawal, and risks reinforcing two of the chief causes of personal difficulties (*kleśas*): ego and misconception. Looking for a father-figure—the need for a transfer relationship—can also be seen in the acceptance of such invitations.

sthānyupanimantraṇe saṅgasmayākaraṇam punaraniṣṭaprasaṅgāt
sthāni-upanimantraṇe saṅga-smaya-akaraṇam punaḥ-aniṣṭa-prasaṅgāt

Sthāni: being, or higher being, having an exalted position. *Upanimantraṇe:* being respectfully invited. *Saṅga:* attachment, pleasure. *Smaya:* wonderment, astonishment. *Akaraṇam:* avoiding. *Punaḥ:* again, once more. *Aniṣṭa:* awful, undesirable. *Prasaṅgāt:* bad leanings, disastrous inclination.

Perfect mastery of the instant and its unfolding brings knowledge born of highly distinctive perception.

Do I tend to use the same replies or solutions over again, or am I incapable of doing the same thing twice?

How can I avoid preconceived ideas, presumptions, or prejudices, and take each instant as new and unique?

What influence does such wisdom have on how I manage my time?

What is the connection between this aphorism and aphorism I.45, which asks about limits to the refining of perception?

To measure the unfolding of time, we use precise units of physical time (hours, minutes, and seconds). This aphorism presents another time unit—the "instant" (*kṣaṇa*) or the smallest unit of time—defined only by the replacement of one characteristic with another. For example, the hand has moved on the clock, my mood is different, and so on. The succession of instants shows that change (*pariṇāma*) has taken place (or not). The flow of time is thus seen differently—according to one's estimation of it. A minute may seem an eternity or quite the opposite. This difference of perception comes from the number of changes seen and whether one likes them or not.

This last type of perfect mastery (*saṁyama*) denotes two spheres: instants defined as such and their succession. One begins to live in the eternal present. There, where there is no distinction, it becomes possible to differentiate even subtleties. All repetition, every stock phrase disappears, whether in the grasp or in the expression: what is seen and said is new and right, adapted to the instant. Like a torch light, such a state of awareness lights up the smallest details.

kṣaṇatatkramayoḥ saṃyamādvivekajaṃ jñānam
kṣaṇa-tat-kramayoḥ saṃyamāt-vivekajaṃ jñānam

Kṣaṇa: the instant. *Tat:* that. *Kramayoḥ:* the unfolding, succession. *Saṃyamāt:* of of perfect concentration. *Viveka:* discernment. *Jaṃ:* being born of. *Jñānam:* knowledge.

III.53

This specific knowledge allows differentiation between two objects otherwise indistinguishable by origin, characteristics, or situation.

Are my powers of observation acute? How can I develop them?

How much does temperament influence shrewd observation?

How can I differentiate between changing perceptions due to the observer's own hesitations and discernment due to wisdom?

How can I reconcile general responses to identical cases with a unique reply for each case?

What qualities are indispensable if we are to risk a new response at each instant?

Does this aphorism mean that a yoga teacher can never give the same reply, nor teach the same type of practice?

Most educational methods are based on grouping similar phenomena: the flu is the flu. However, according to this aphorism and indeed for certain types of medicine, no two strains of flu are alike, even for a given person. At this high level of perception, it becomes impossible to give the same reply to apparently identical situations. Like the parents of twins, the slightest sign permits differentiation.

Apparent similarity has three sources: similarity due to birth; similarity of characteristics within a given species; and lastly, similarity of place—geographical situation—in which the thing or being evolves.

When perception is refined, similarity, uniformity, and boredom disappear. Being present in every instant gives an ever-sparkling attraction to existence and enables one to distinguish it from Essence.

jātilakṣaṇadeśairanyatānavacchedāttulyayostataḥ pratipattiḥ
jāti-lakṣaṇa-deśaiḥ-anyatā-anavacchedāt-tulyayoḥ-tataḥ pratipattiḥ

Jāti: birth, class, caste. *Lakṣaṇa:* characteristic. *Deśaiḥ:* place, situation. *Anyatā:* difference. *Anavacchedāt:* because of the absence of distinction (or distinguishing mark). *Tulyayoḥ:* of two similar things. *Tataḥ:* then. *Pratipattiḥ:* discriminating knowledge, distinction.

III.54

**Such is knowledge born of discrimination—
it flows spontaneously and pertains to
any object, at any level.**

Is my attitude usually the right one? Are my remarks and responses appropriate?

Does this aphorism infer that such a person no longer hesitates and that he or she can reply to any question at any moment?

Does such an elevated view entail growing nearer to, or growing away from, others?

What sort of prudence goes with this elevated knowledge?

The spontaneity, correctness of view, and precise replies of an experienced scholar are often limited to his or her speciality. From the wise one, however, accurate global knowledge spontaneously flows, with no casting about for it or asking a question. Such knowledge can cover any object, at any level, in any shape.

The replies from such a one do not depend on the sum of knowledge received and stored up. The inner being expresses itself through a transparent personality.

tārakaṃ sarvaviṣayaṃ sarvathāviṣayamakramaṃ ceti vivekajaṁ jñānam

tārakaṃ sarvaviṣayaṃ sarvathāviṣayam-akramaṃ ca-iti vivekajaṃ jñānam

Tārakam: transcendental, liberating, spontaneous. *Sarvaviṣayam:* for any, all object(s). *Sarvathāviṣayam:* for any form of object, that is to say, at every level. *Akramam:* without seeking to do so, without taking steps. *Ca:* and. *Iti:* such is. *Viveka:* discrimination. *Jam:* being born of. *Jñānam:* knowledge.

III.55

When the purity of the peaceful mind is identical with that of the spiritual entity, that is liberation.

What is my degree of inner liberty?

What parts do the radiance of joy and peace play in this appreciation?

How can I be both completely independent and liberated, yet also respectful of others and of social and cultural pressures?

Do purity and mental transparency mean that the personality is colorless and without temperament?

Is there such a thing as a gratuitous act?

Is there a connection between this aphorism and aphorism I.41 which illustrates the contemplative state, using the diamond as an example?

Liberation corresponds to a state of freedom—of independence that does not consist in fleeing the world, but in blooming in it, as much with others as alone.

At this high level, the personality no longer distorts perceptions, words, or actions, because the mental function is colorless—transparent.

There is no longer the slightest attachment even to a good cause because there is no association with the world.

For all who live in this world, being in full bloom gives rise to the consideration that "they are not of the world, just as I am not of the world" as the Evangelist so rightly puts it.*

sattvapuruṣayoḥ śuddhisāmye kaivalyam
sattva-puruṣayoḥ śuddhi-sāmye kaivalyam

Sattva: the state of peace. *Puruṣayoḥ:* the spiritual entity. *Śuddhi:* pure. *Sāmye:* identical, equal. *Kaivalyam:* serenity, liberation, beatitude.

*St John 17:16.

CHAPTER IV

Serenity

kaivalyapādaḥ

SERENITY

What does the word "liberation" evoke in me?

Can I make it my objective?

Is such an objective stimulating or discouraging?

The Sanskrit word, kaivalyapādaḥ (serenity), also means independence or isolation. Does this mean few persons reach this state?

Chapter IV describes the culmination of human evolution and the functioning of the human psyche in such a state. This is the state of serenity, or spiritual liberation.

In answering the following questions, this chapter also describes how an individual in this state of radiance may influence others, and it precisely sets out the situation of a liberated person.

IV.1	Where do exceptional faculties come from?
IV.2 to IV.8	What is the human psyche?
IV.9 to IV.26	In light of yoga, what is the nature of human being, our relationship to life, and the quality of spiritual liberation we can attain?
IV.27 to IV.28	What can we do if we lose this state of liberation?
IV.29 to IV.34	What is ultimate liberation?

kaivalyapādaḥ
kaivalya-pādaḥ

Kaivalya: serenity, beatitude, liberation. *Pādaḥ:* chapter, foot, quarter.

IV.1

Superior faculties originate from birth, the use of consecrated plants, recitation of mantra, ascetic discipline, and contemplation.

How can one born with powers avoid using them for personal gain?

How can I make sure I use consecrated plants correctly?

In practicing mantra, how can I let go of excessive attachment to this means or to the one who handed it down?

Does all self-discipline impede social life?

How can one bloom using these means?

Is patience a key to the use of these superior means and contemplation?

Do I have enough patience?

The first source of these faculties, birth, is different from the others, because there is no way of obtaining this source, and it is extremely rare. Hindus attribute it to benefits acquired from previous lives. Some believers believe it is due to divine grace. Received spontaneously and not as the result of undertakings during this life, such faculties are fragile and can be wasted. The fragility of this state is like that of the spoiled son of a rich family. Not having had to struggle to conquer and defend his riches, he risks being easy prey to envious foes, as well as succumbing to his own bad leanings.

Ingesting certain plants can also bring about these faculties, not because of their aphrodisiac qualities, but because they have been consecrated during rituals that confer a particular power on them. Using an element exterior to the body, however, can give rise to attachment to the ritual.

Mantra is a divine word or sacred formula that can be one or more syllables or parts, pronounced aloud, murmured or spoken mentally, or linked to breathing or not. One receives a *mantra* from an inspired master. Its efficacy is linked to the intensity of the discipline of the one who hands it on. Its elaboration and transmission obey precise rules as presented in classical treatises. Many cultures use *mantra.* Their recitation should be distinguished from prayer; mantra is a higher way than gifts of birth or ingesting consecrated plants.

Ascetic discipline, as a means to acquiring superior powers, involves purification and elimination of all obstacles. Several ways with different effects are possible: discipline with sleep, food, continence, donations, practice, truth, and so on. It is a powerful means, but if overdone, it can harm the body.

Contemplation here encompasses the whole of the yoga of eight limbs (II.29). It offers the advantage of a well-balanced way of proceeding, making a place for all levels of being and is relatively certain. Results come about little by little as personal obstacles are overcome, so there is less risk of backsliding.

The order of the five methods is therefore a hierarchical one, contemplation being superior to all the others.

janmaoṣadhimantratapaḥ samādhijāḥ siddhayaḥ
janma-oṣadhi-mantra-tapaḥ samādhi-jāḥ siddhayaḥ

Janma: birth. *Oṣadhi:* herbs, plants consumed during a sacred ritual. *Mantra:* sacred formula. *Tapaḥ:* ascetic discipline. *Samādhḥ:* contemplation. *Jāḥ:* born of. *Siddhayaḥ:* powers, higher faculties.

IV.2

Positive evolution is the result of one's innermost nature.

How can it help me to know that inwardly I already possess all that is necessary to develop and improve myself?

What are the limits to my potential?

Does this road to autonomy present only positive aspects?

Once having done away with excessive inertia (tamas*), as well as too much change* (rajas*), what part does time play in reaching equilibrium and radiance* (sattva*)?*

Lavoisier's idea that "Nothing is lost, nothing is created, all is transformed," illustrates this aphorism well. Each form of life, as well as each human being, is a physical entity that holds within itself the whole program of its evolution and elevation. In short, evolution is a natural phenomenon.

This viewpoint differs from the religious precept that all proceeds from God. Being aware of possibilities contained within fosters responsibility and reinforces confidence in one's own capacities.

Evolution occurs at every level—physical, emotional, mental, and spiritual. Such mutations take place within the domain of the constituent qualities of nature (*guṇa-s*).

Degrees of evolution correspond to successive adjustments, transformations, and eliminations, rather than to what one acquires.

jātyantarapariṇāmaḥ prakṛtypūrāt
jāti-antara-pariṇāmaḥ prakṛti-apūrāt

Jāti: birth, class, caste, race, specific character. *Antara:* inner, interior, near, contained. *Pariṇāma:* evolution, change, mutation. *Prakṛti:* tangible nature, matter. prt: filling oneself completely, pour, fill.

The causes of evolution do not set nature in motion, but withdraw obstacles, like a gardener opening an irrigation canal.

How can this aphorism help me with personal, and professional relationships?

Which obstacles in my own personality (kleśas) interfere with my truly helping others?

Does the word "cause" refer to the guide's intelligence, to technical elements handed down, or to the action of the one who is evolving?

Is there a connection between this aphorism and detachment from the fruits of action (karma-yoga, vairāgya)?

Although nature is self-evolving (IV.2), obstacles can diminish and even stop evolution. Everything in us is made for change, but obstacles block us so that we need outside intervention in order to modify our nature. A catalyst indirectly withdraws impediments just as a gardener removes obstacles from an irrigation canal so the water can flow freely on its own.

A human catalyst, when helping another, does not give anything the other does not already hold within. Through helping others this way, we gain insight into our own problems. We need this know-how.

Irrigation has to respect natural forces. The primary role of a teacher, parent, or business director is to create favorable conditions in which others can come into fulfillment and give their best. We cannot and should not take another's place nor bear another's burdens. Aphorisms IV.2 and this one are complementary and are very useful in active life.

nimittamaprayojakaṃ prakṛtīnāṃ varaṇabhedastu tataḥ kṣetrikavat

nimittam-aprayojakaṃ prakṛtīnāṃ varaṇa-bhedaḥ-tu tataḥ kṣetrika-vat

Nimittam: cause, reason. *Aprayojakam:* inoperative. *Prakṛtīnām:* of nature. *Varaṇa:* dyke, rampart. *Bhedaḥ:* boring, piercing, breaking (open). *Tu:* but. *Tataḥ:* then, following, after. *Kṣetrikavat:* like a gardener.

IV.4

Individual consciousness develops only in contact with another individual consciousness.

What qualities must I develop to truly appreciate the way others, such as parents and teachers, have influenced me?

Can I refuse to see these influences?

What would the consequences be?

Can I overestimate the influence of certain people on me?

How can I become more aware of my influence over others?

Can I refuse it or become even more blind to it?

Is this influence limited to mental function alone, or can it affect the body, health, and destiny?

Where does judicious influence end and manipulation begin?

Aphorisms IV.2 and IV.3 explain how individual consciousness evolves toward liberation. Its source is presented here. Though potentially present in everybody, it can develop only through contact with another radiant individual consciousness.

Such a mode of growth is seen not only in the way young people identify with matinée "idols," but also in the influence of great spiritual masters, which transcends time and space.

This aphorism takes account of the structural relationship in which a human being is fulfilled. It is a network of infinitely complex influences that are difficult, even impossible, to know completely, in terms of influences both received and given—for example, parents' love for their child, a teacher's attention to the student, friendship toward a friend, and so on.

Without a strong personality, there is no influence; and without detachment from one's personality, no correct influence.

nirmāṇa-cittāni-asmitā-mātrāt
nirmāṇacittānyasmitāmātrāt

Nirmāṇa: measure, influence. *Cittāni:* spirits. *Asmitā:* individual consciousness, "I am," ego. *Mātrāt:* because it consists essentially in, only coming from.

A single individual consciousness is operative over many others in varied manifestations.

What or who has been my primary model? Why?

How have I experienced its influence?

Am I still blind with admiration or in reactive opposition?

How do I control or refuse anothers influence when necessary?

Do others imitate me?

What is the role of imitation, as proposed by some religions, in a person's spiritual evolution?

This aphorism develops and clarifies the results of the preceding one. The more someone is calm, lucid, or rich, the more people he or she will influence. Like a high mountaintop seen from afar, one's radiance can cut across the centuries. It is this way for great spiritual masters.

An image or word perceived by a crowd of people affects each one differently. As T. K. V. Desikachar says: "The same fall of rain can relieve a peasant in the throes of a drought, make a mother with no correct shelter for her child anxious, and have no effect on the vast ocean."

pravṛttibhede prayojakaṃ cittamekamanekeṣām
pravṛtti-bhede prayojakaṃ cittam-ekam-anekeṣām

Pravṛtti: manifestation, activity. *Bhede:* cut, separation, division. *Prayojakam:* efficacious, operative. *Cittam:* the psyche, the mind, thought. *Ekam:* one only, single. *Anekeṣām:* over many others, many, a lot.

IV.6

Then, that which arises from meditation produces no negative influence over others.

Do I influence others from the meditative state?

How can I recognize when the person influencing me is in that state?

How can I encourage this state so that others receive correct influence?

Why does Patañjali advise meditation, the seventh limb of yoga, and not contemplation, the eighth?

Do several influences favor evolution simultaneously?

How do contradictory influences affect a person?

Can one experience positive influence in the professional field and negative influence in the family or vice-versa?

It was stated earlier that individual consciousness awakens only through contact with another consciousness, and that strong personalities influence many individuals. Patañjali lists the different kinds of influences. If the guide is in a meditative state, and at the same time concentrating on and linked to the object of concentration—the child, disciple, or student—the influence is positive. When the guide appreciates the receiver's capacities, no anxiety, fear, or suffering can appear in the one influencing or in the receiver.

The word *dhyāna* here not only means meditation, but also "reflection." This aphorism reminds us of the need to reflect before, during, and after action and to be aware of ourselves in the relationship with a guide. It also means "prayer." A believer will first pray. The more significant an action, the more one must ponder and pray.

The quality of the influence depends on the three constituent qualities of nature (*guṇas*): It will be correct when equilibrium and clarity (*sattva*) predominate, and incorrect when over-activity (*rajas*) and heaviness (*tamas*) predominate.

According to the commentary of *Vyāsa,* meditation, contemplation, and the yoga of eight limbs as means are superior to gifts of birth, ingesting plants, reciting mantra, and ascetic discipline.

tatra dhyānajamanāśayam
tatra dhyāna-jam-anāśayam

Tatra: there. *Dhyāna:* meditation, reflection. *Jam:* arise from, be born of. *Anāśayam:* absence of negative influences, of latency.

**The yogi's action is neither black nor white;
the action of others is of three kinds.**

Do I tend toward black, or injudicious, acts or do I wish to do as much good for others as for myself?

Is there a connection between these tendencies and obstacles in the personality (II.3)?

Is recognizing what is at the root of the personality enough to diminish such tendencies?

Is there such a thing as a gratuitous act?

The desire to replace injudicious actions with judicious, or "white," ones may seem obvious, but how does one move beyond both—beyond good and evil? What can this bring?

The action of the yogi, an individual in a meditative state (IV.6), is judicious. Negative tendencies in the personality of the yogi neither engender nor influence his or her action. A yogi does not make promises he or she cannot keep, but gives only what is good in order to do good, with no thought of receiving direct or indirect benefit.

Two things can be given: the impulse, or energy, through describing and enhancing the aim, and the choice of steps to take, by clarifying the starting point. Any thought, word, or gesture toward another that covers any more ground than this is a good action with negative results.

The yogi's action, whatever the origin of his or her faculties, is, therefore, neither good, nor bad, nor mixed—it is judicious, or correct. What is difficult is to remain in this state, despite outside influences. One should always remind oneself of a person's best qualities and remain careful. The action of those who are not yogis can be black, white, or, as is often the case, a mixture of the two.

karmāśuklākṛṣṇaṃ yoginastrividhamitareṣām
karma-aśukla-akṛṣṇaṃ yoginaḥ-trividham-itareṣām

Karma: action, act, work. *Aśukla:* nonluminous, without brilliance or shine, not white, not positive. *Akṛṣṇaṃ:* not somber, not black, not negative. *Yoginaḥ:* in the case of, for a yogi. *Trividham:* of three kinds. *Itareṣām:* in the case of others, in others.

IV.8

Consequences surely follow these inappropriate tendencies.

Are my own erroneous tendencies sufficiently few to allow me to accept responsibilities? How can I know?

What should I do when I realize I am acting inappropriately?

To rid myself of improper manifestations, should I play them down or face them?

What are the risks of provoking their appearance in myself and in others?

Unless we sufficiently reduce our own personal problems, as our influence over others grows, we place them and ourselves in danger. In effect, as soon as circumstances allow, we see the resurgence of our erroneous tendencies. The higher we are, the more painful others' suffering and our own fall will be.

It is not just incorrect action that causes suffering; actions that are good to excess and those that are mixed, where it is difficult to distinguish the good from the bad, cause suffering as well.

Erroneous tendencies do not necessarily diminish simply because light has been thrown on them. Intensive work on the personality and gradual evolution due to practicing the eight limbs of yoga will surely do away with these obstacles more than any of the other means presented in aphorism IV.1.

The word *vāsana,* which Patañjali chose to designate these latent tendencies is a synonym of the word *saṃskāra.* But, generally, *vāsana* designates what is innate and *saṃskāra* what is acquired. *Vāsana* here, however, represents these innate and acquired tendencies as a whole.

tatastadvipākānuguṇānāmevābhivyaktirvāsanānām
tataḥ tad-vipāka-anuguṇānām-abhivyaktiḥ-vāsanānām

Tataḥ: it follows that. *Tad:* that. *Vipāka:* result, consequence or effect, fruit. *Anuguṇānām:* appropriate to. *Eva:* in truth, certainly. *Abhivyaktiḥ:* manifestation. *Vāsanānām:* latent tendencies.

Despite differences in birth, place, and era, our behavior continually perpetuates itself because of the unity of form between memory and mental permeation.

Is my behavior more or less stereotyped? Why?

What qualities can help me recognize my conditioning and rid myself of it, if necessary?

Do we have only the freedom we allow ourselves?

Why is it so difficult to accept or allow change while staying with one's immediate family (the snake hides itself away when sloughing, doesn't it)?

Why is this so even when we substitute a more comfortable way of behaving for a painful one?

How does memory influence latent impressions and vice versa? What conclusions should we draw?

In this aphorism, Patañjali begins to address the problem presented in aphorism IV.8 by explaining how latent and subconscious impressions (mental permeation) work. He offers a solution in aphorism IV.11.

Our thought presents itself as a coherent whole. Our mental function is so perfected that it ensures this coherence by calling on elements that spring from various sources: innate behavior and attitudes resulting from our experiences or recent information. Thus, our actions and our behavior result from a chain of causes and effects that reaches back to the beginning of time. The consequences are alternating moments of joy and pain (II.14).

Our behavior is thus induced by memory, which corresponds to thought, psychic permeation, and functional structure, even before we are conscious of it.

jātideśakālavyavahitānāmapyānantaryaṃ
smṛtisaṃskārayohekarūpatvāt
jāti-deśa-kāla-vyavahitānām-api-ānantaryaṃ
smṛti-saṃskārayoḥ-eka-rūpatvāt

Jāti: birth, caste, type, rank. *Deśa:* space, place. *Kāla:* time. *Vyavahitānām:* separated. *Api:* even. nantaryam: continuity, simultaneity. *Smṛti:* memory. *Saṃskāryo:* mental permeation. *Ekarūpatvāt:* because of similarity, of uniformity.

IV.10

The desire for life is eternal, therefore, mental permeation has no origin.

Am I aware of desire? Am I slave to it?

What can awareness that desire is permanent bring us?

How can we solve the problems desire poses?

Is it easier to stop desire or to sublimate it (I.37)?

How can a better understanding of desire influence our relationships?

How do giving and receiving satisfy or strengthen desire, or give rise to irrational behavior?

How can one have a burning interest as a motive, yet be detached from the result?

How are desire, attachment (II.7), and fear (II.9) related?

The life impulse corresponds to multitudinous forms of desire: desire for material or other goods, desire for recognition, desire to satisfy affective, sensual, and sexual impulses, and to raise oneself spiritually. This life force, inherent in life itself, is present in all of life's kingdoms, like a plant attracted by the light. It is at the root of any motive based on the hope of benefit and is strengthened by giving, as well as refusing. It is one of the keys to human relationships, and as this desire springs eternal, we should not rejoice too quickly, thinking we have passed this stage. Even if we see nothing negative for some time, it remains latent. Only circumstances can prevent the return of these problems. Nevertheless, one should never give up hope. Even when faced with serious illness, one is still inhabited by the desire of physiological, psychological, and spiritual evolution. Don't rejoice too quickly, but never despair! Be vigilant!

tāsāmanāditvaṃ cāśiṣo nityatvāt
tāsām anāditvaṃ ca-āśiṣaḥ nityatvāt

Tāsām: of them (negative mental imprints, IV.8) *Anāditvam:* without origin. *Ca:* and. *Āśiṣaḥ:* instinct of survival, need for possession. *Nityatvāt:* because of the eternal nature of, permanent.

Cause, consequence, mental coloring, and object support are interdependent, and when they disappear, desire ceases to manifest.

What objects hamper me?

What impulses give rise to attachment to these objects?

Are there less harmful objects toward which I could turn such impulses?

In this kind of work, where does progressiveness come in?

What is the relationship between this aphorism and aphorisms I.12, I.37, and II.3?

The basic impulse of desire shows itself progressively in a chain of causes and effects. First, it appears as a cause, with one or more erroneous impulses of the personality (*kleśas*). Whether we are aware or not of this impulse of desire, it is very difficult to stop it.

Thereafter, this tendency in the personality has, as a consequence, a relationship more or less marked by attachment or detachment with regard to using certain sense organs. On a third level, clarity or mental confusion appear as characteristics of the individual. This ends in fixation on a precise action or object.

Let us go back link by link. Drinking alcohol stimulates attachment to a psychic and digestive sensation that obscures any clear sight of the consequences of the act, and engenders a general lack of mental clarity. Getting rid of an alcoholic drink in one's surroundings is only one of the elements that can liberate us from the desire. Though getting rid of an object is generally the first stage, it does not suffice, for example, one can continue to suffer from desire for a departed person.

As Vyāsa puts it: "From a cause like virtue, pleasure or happiness result; from impiety, pain or misery; from happiness, attachment; and from misery, hatred. From attachment and hatred, effort results; and from effort, action in the form of mental and bodily movements or words. Thus, creatures benefit or injure others and from this arise piety and impiety, happiness and misery, attachment and hatred. Thus the six-spoked wheel of birth and rebirth (worldliness) revolves constantly. The motivating powers of this perpetually moving wheel are ignorance and ingratitude, which are at the root of all misery."

hetuphalāśrayālambanaiḥ saṅgṛhītatvādeṣāmabhāve tadabhāvaḥ
hetu-phala-āśraya-ālambanaiḥ saṅgṛhītatvāt-eṣām-abhāve
tad-abhāvaḥ

Hetu: cause, motive. *Phala:* fruit, result, consequence. *Āśraya:* mental coloring. *Ālambanaḥi:* the support, the staying point, base. *Saṅgrhītatvāt:* given the seizure, grasp. *Eṣām:* of these latter. *Abhāve*: in the absence of. *Tad:* that. *Abhāvaḥ:* absence.

The past and the future are always potentially present. Their manifestations depend on individual and universal laws as a whole.

What can I learn from knowing that my past and my future are always present in me? Is it a hopeful or an unhopeful sign?

Does never believing a problem is solved give rise more to prudence or to fear?

Does thinking that "while there is life, there is hope" produce optimism or illusion in me?

How does the study of this aphorism influence my attitude toward my past and toward my potential?

What is the connection between this aphorism and:
- *detachment from the results of action (I.15)?*
- *evolution (III.9 to III.12)?*

This aphorism continues the theme of the preceding one, adding the notion of time. Water, for example, can be ice or steam depending on the temperature. Its state, always a provisional one, is ordered by natural laws of physics and chemistry.

All states of mind, all difficulties, and all kinds of old, erroneous behavior are engraved in us and ready to appear again if circumstances allow. Similarly, the whole of our future is there in a potential state. Depending on circumstances, these potentialities show up more or less rapidly. We should never believe that a problem is definitely settled—quite simply it does not show anymore. But also,we should never forget hope.

The past remains present in us through the sentiments it aroused; the future is present through our potential, our hopes, and our thoughts. If we tend to paint our past and our future, only the present appears under its true colors. The essential thing is, therefore, to live in the present.

atītānāgataṃ svarūpato 'styadhvabhedāddharmāṇām
atīta-anāgataṃ svarūpataḥ-asti-adhva-bhedāt-dharmāṇām

Atīta: the past. *Anāgatam:* the future. *Svarūpataḥ:* his (its, her) own essential form. *Asti:* is. *Adhva-bhedāt:* at different moments. *Dharmāṇām:* the laws, the properties, the universal order, destiny.

Whether individual and universal laws manifest or not depends on the three constituent qualities of nature.

Depending on the needs of the day, am I easily influenced by inertia (tamas), overactivity (rajas), or clarity (sattva)?

Is one of these qualities predominant in me? If so, which one?

Is it more a help or a hindrance?

What quality helps prevent a relapse into past insomnia, by favoring maintenance of present stability?

What are the connections between this aphorism and aphorisms II.18 and II.19 with regard to qualities (śilam) and their manifestation?

The main systems of Hindu thought all say that nature manifests itself through three qualities: inertia (*tamas*), overactivity (*rajas*), clarity (*sattva*). Our mental coloring is what results, at a given moment, from these three primary qualities (see commentary on I.16).

Depending on how open or clear the mind is, how understanding (*sattva*), how active or changeable (*rajas*), how limited or obtuse (*tamas*)—these characteristics show more or less. The same word, the same sentence, can bring the past back to the reader or lead him or her toward new realities, depending on his or her characteristics.

This notion of constituent qualities of nature is difficult, even impossible, to understand. In thinking we have understood, certainly we understood nothing as we seek to grasp the intrinsic nature of the instrument of perception by using it. That is why it has been stated in the *Śāstras:* "The ultimate nature of the *guṇas* is never visible; what is seen is extremely ephemeral, like an illusion," (*Vyāsa*).

te vyaktasūkṣmā guṇātmānaḥ
te vyakta-sūkṣmāḥ guṇa-ātmānaḥ

Te: they (the laws). *Vyakta:* manifested, of the realm of effect. *Sūkṣmāḥ:* subtle, unmanifested, causal. *Guṇa:* the constituent qualities of nature. *Ātmānaḥ:* have the value, the nature, the qualities of.

An object's reality depends on uniting the changes of the three constituent qualities of nature.

What image of myself do I show others?

What produces my coherence?

How has this coherence developed and where is it going?

How can I discern the factors in my personality that are most susceptible to change?

Is changing my diet or surroundings, for example, a cause or a result of evolution?

Can I make decisions without being clear about a situation?

Can I have solid judgment, yet be ready to throw it into the balance?

An object's reality is always a specific state in continual evolution. All perception is provisional and instantaneous, that is, it is real, but reduced, with regard to the ever-changing universe.

In short, the three constituent qualities of nature manifest as perceptions received by an instrument that is itself made up of these three qualities. This instrument is influenced as well when it perceives the object.

This means that any conclusion is provisional. As soon as one pronounces it, it is already out of date—a mere stage. It is, therefore, imprudent to conclude, judge, or fix an opinion on an event or an individual.

Any situation can evolve, even if our conditioning puts a brake on any changes. Far too often, our desperate efforts to present a coherent picture to others keep us from evolving in a way that is positive and desirable, when, really, anything is possible.

pariṇāmaikatvātvastutattvam
pariṇāma-ekatvāt-vastu-tattvam

Pariṇāma: transformation, evolution, change. *Ekatvāt:* the state of being one, of unity. *Vastu:* object, basic reality, concrete. *Tattvam:* quintessence, essential reality.

IV.15

The psyche's fragmentary nature creates a divergence between the object and one's grasp of it, even though the object itself remains coherent.

Is the way I see things usually positive or negative?

Does this aphorism mean that the other is right, that I am right, or that both of us are right?

What impact does understanding this aphorism have on respect for another?

If every perception differs, what is absolute truth (I.48)?

How can I become aware of my subjectivity and lessen it?

Are all opinions at once both true and complementary?

In a group, should we exclude a person with a different opinion or, rather, take notice of him or her?

What is the connection between this aphorism and aphorism II.19 (multiplicity of manifestation)?

An observer perceives the same object differently depending on his or her state of mind. In fact, this aphorism has at least two meanings: two people perceive the same object differently; and one person perceives the same object differently at two different moments. Seen by virtue, it appears pleasing; by vice, painful; by stupidity, silly; and by the wise person, in its intrinsic reality.

The mind perceives an object—made up essentially of the constituent qualities of nature—because that object interests the mind. This interest colors perception, which, consequently, is rarely objective. For example, a monument is a means of subsistence for the keeper, an object of curiosity for the tourist, a witness of the past for the historian, and a model for the architect. We must, therefore, dilute this coloring by studying the self and, in the yoga tradition, by learning to chant in a dual relationship (*II.1, svādhyāya*).

vastusāmye cittabhedāttayorvibhaktaḥ panthāḥ
vastu-sāmye citta-bhedāt-tayoḥ-vibhaktaḥ panthāḥ

Vastu: object. *Sāmye:* identical, equal. *Citta:* mind, mental function, thought. *Bhedāt:* because of the fragmentary nature, division. *Tayoḥ:* of these two. *Vibhaktaḥ:* distinction, divergence. *Panthāḥ:* paths.

For an object to exist, the mind need not perceive it. Otherwise, without perception, would there be any objective reality?

Is my view of the world:

- *created by my mind?*
- *an illusory reality?*
- *an evolving reality?*

To what extent can this aphorism modify:

- *my perception of things in general?*
- *my perception of difficulties peculiar to me?*
- *my perception of others' difficulties?*

*If a yoga teacher affirms that the world is illusion (*maya*), does this respect the point of view of the discipline he represents?*

What bearing does this viewpoint have on a rational and non-abstract student?

How does the yoga viewpoint, which affirms the world's reality, influence the evolution of those who adhere to a rationalist practice?

Patañjali here specifies the philosopher's view of the world, whose reality he affirms. All objects are real, perceived or not. This point of view refutes other systems, such as Buddhism for which a perceived object is more a product of the mind, or the *Advaïta Vedanta,* which states that the object's existence is fictitious.

The philosopher's assertion determines the attitude to the world and, in particular, how to approach a problem and solve it.

Whatever difficulty someone exposes, whether it is a figment of the imagination or not, yoga recognizes it as something real. That enables us to listen to others at the level of their difficulties. To solve them, the approach then consists in replacing this reality with another less harmful one. The solution in other systems, on the contrary, resides more in trying to stop mental output or in becoming aware of the unreal character of the object perceived.

For example, Granddad promises a reward to his granddaughter for doing something. When she accomplishes this act, Granddad has forgotten the amount promised and gives her only half, so she is upset about it. We can envisage different approaches to the situation. Some pretend that this suffering comes from the false hopes produced by her mind and that the solution then lies in waking up to its unreal character. For a yogi, the expectation of the reward is real, but must be replaced by a second reality—that of the diminished reward. Suffering comes from the difficulty in accepting the change. And suffering disappears when one understands the causes of this resistance to the change and its acceptance.

na caikacittatantraṃ cedvastu tadapramāṇakaṃ tad kiṃ syāt
na ca-eka-citta-tantraṃ cet-vastu tad-apramāṇakaṃ tad kiṃ syāt

Na: no, not. *Ca:* and. *Eka:* single, alone. *Citta:* the psyche, the mind. *Tantram:* depending on. *Cet:* if. *Vastu:* object. *Tad:* that (refering to *citta*). *Apramāṇakaṃ:* that which is only. *Tadā:* then (afterwards). *Kiṃ:* is…? How? *Syāt:* would be.

The mind perceives objects or not, depending on the attraction they exert and the interest one has in them.

How attracted am I to others and to life in general?

What attracts me most?

What interests me most?

Does this aphorism apply mostly to family, profession, friendship, or others?

How can this aphorism prevent us from manipulating others?

Does it enable us to modulate a transference relationship? How?

How can this aphorism enhance our human relationships?

What are the connections between this aphorism and the notions of attachment (II.7), repulsion (II.8), and detachment (I.15)?

This aphorism essentially deals with human relationships. We perceive an object under two conditions: the first is the attraction it exerts over us, and the second is the degree to which we invest ouselves in the relationship. These two links can vary in intensity, from their absence to their maximum strength.

For a given individual another person is an object, and their relationship takes place through four channels whose power can be modified.

1. The first channel is the desire *A* feels when confronted with *B* (*uparāga*).
2. The second is *A's* wish to invest or not in the relationship with *B* (*apekṣi*).
3. The third is the desire *B* feels when faced with *A* (*uparāga*).
4. The fourth is *B's* wish to invest or not in the relationship with *A* (*apekṣi*).

Both people involved can directly influence two channels. *A* can modulate will and attention toward *B* (channel 2), and strengthen or reduce the attraction *B* feels (channel 3). In the same way, *B* can work with channels 4 and 1. In this way, we can build or destroy our human relationships.

We can separate ourselves from an object, if it is a source of problems, even by momentarily turning the attention toward another object.

To see our way clearly in a relationship, we can ask four questions:

1. Am I attracted to the other person?
2. Am I ready to invest in the relationship?
3. Is this other person attracted to me?
4. Is this other ready to invest in the relationship?

If we want to help someone become free of a dependency or a destructive pleasure, we could draw his or her attention toward a less harmful pleasure by making it attractive and encouraging redirected interest.

This aphorism speaks about being able to reinforce or leave a relationship depending on needs. This ability must be very solid when it becomes necessary to speak of certain basic truths to another. We must be able to drop a relationship when it has become harmful or worn out.

To resume, depending on yoga:

- The object is real; so is the mind;
- The object is not the same as the mind.
- The object is multiple, and the mind is multiple;
- Both the object and the mind always change, therefore, the relationship between them changes as well.

taduparāgpekṣitvāccittasya vastu jñātājñātam
tad-uparāga-apekṣitvāt cittasya vastu jñāta-ajñātam

Tad: of that (*vastu:* the object). *Uparāga:* influence, attractiveness, coloration. *Apekitvāt:* because of the gaze placed on, investment in the relationship. *Cittasya*: of the mind, the psyche. *Vastu:* the object. *Jñāta:* perceived, known. *Ajñātam:* unperceived, not perceived, unknown, not known.

The spiritual entity is unchanging and always knows and is master of the ever-changing mind.

Is it difficult to accept a superior dimension in me? If so, why?

Do my behavior and my choices respect that inner presence in myself and in others?

What qualities can help me to recognize that dimension and its superiority?

How can I develop awareness of this?

What have I learned in life? By asking this, how will my daily life change?

Why does the yoga tradition assert that words can only lead us to an idea, and that to go beyond words, a teacher is necessary?

What is the connection between this aphorism, aphorism I.20, and the next aphorism?

This aphorism has several meanings: There is something other than the mind, and this other reality is its ever-perceiving master. Our mind may seem to see things, but it does not itself really perceive, it is the spiritual entity that perceives. Whatever our degree of lucidity or self-complacency, we have an eyewitness inside—nothing escapes it. We should devote our whole lives to letting it shine through. The spiritual entity is an unchangeable, permanent, eternal reference point that allows perception of change.

A famous *Upaniṣad "dṛg dṛśya viveka"* (discernment between the perceiving entity and the perceived) demonstrates this point of view clearly.

I. The form is perceived and the eye is its perceiver. It (eye) is perceived and the mind is its perceiver. The mind with its modifications is perceived and the Witness (the Self) is verily the perceiver. But It (the Witness) is not perceived (by any other).

II. The forms (objects of perception) appear various because of such distinctions as blue, yellow, gross, subtle, short, long, and so on.

III. Such characteristics of the eye as blindness, sharpness, or dullness, the mind can follow because it is a unity. This also applies to (whatever is perceived through) the ear, skin, and so on.

IV. Consciousness illuminates (such other mental states as) desire, determination and doubt, belief and nonbelief, constancy and its opposite, modesty, understanding, fear, and others, because it (Consciousness) is a unity.

V. This Consciousness neither rises nor sets. It does not increase; nor does it suffer decay. Being self-luminous, it illuminates everything else without any other aid.

The spiritual being is superior to the mind, and recognizing this dimension entirely modifies an individual's values and choices in life. Through this we find out what lies beyond words, or mental activity. Never to be content with words is, therefore, desirable.

sadā jñātāścittavṛttayastatprabhoḥ puruṣasyāpariṇāmitvāt
sadā jñātāḥ-citta-vṛttayaḥ-tat-prabhoḥ
puruṣasya-apariṇāmitvāt

Sadā: always, unceasingly. *Jñātāḥ:* known. *Citta:* the psyche, the mind. *Vṛttayḥa:* fluctuations. *Tat:* that. *Prabhoḥ:* master, lord. *Puruṣasya:* of the spiritual entity. *Apariṇāmitvāt:* because of an unevolving state.

The mind cannot perceive itself as object.

To what extent does my mind influence or faithfully carry out my decisions?

Is the reply different depending on the action?

If my mind distorts reality too much, what should I do?

What qualities do I need to recognize that my mind has no awareness of itself?

What are the main obstacles to this awakening of consciousness?

What can it bring me, and how will it affect my relationships?

If our mind, which belongs to the material world, is not itself aware, why do we grant it so much importance?

This aphorism finishes defining the perceiving entity, the object perceived, and their relationships.

We find it difficult to acknowledge that our mind is not at all aware of itself. Patañjali asserts this here by using the word for light and splendor (*bhās*)—our mind has no light of its own. Light has two powers: it shines and it illuminates other things, that is, it makes objects appear. The source of light or consciousness does not spring from the mind. A server who brings a dish receives compliments or reproaches even though the server has nothing to do with it—the artisan is the cook. In the same way we attribute a role to our mind that it does not possess. Like a mirror, it produces an image of a perception for which it is only a more or less faithful instrument. As Vyāsa points out: "But mind is knowable because, from a reflection of the action in one's mind, people are seen to experience tendencies such as 'I am angry,' 'I am afraid,' 'I like it.' This would not be possible unless there is cognition of what is happening in one's own mind."

na tatsvābhāsaṃ dṛśyatvāt
na tat-svābhāsaṃ dṛśyatvāt

Na: and no, not. *Tat:* that (refers to *cittam,* IV.18). *Svābhāsam*: its own sparkle, brilliance. *Dṛśyatvāt:* being perceived.

IV.20

And it is impossible to be conscious of the two simultaneously.

What are the roles of observing my mind and using it in my daily life?

How can I go from one level to another?

When is it preferable to look at the mind instead of taking action?

Where and how does yoga practice fit here?

What is the connection between this aphorism and the expression "examine one's conscience"?

Must I spend my whole life examining my conscience? What are the consequences?

If it is impossible simultaneously to act and to see oneself in the act, how can we understand the saying: "Think before, during, and after the action"?

Two important notions were just presented in aphorisms IV.18 and IV.19: There exists an unchanging, higher spiritual entity, ever-conscious of the mind; and, the mind itself has no consciousness. Patañjali makes it clear here that one cannot be conscious simultaneously of the mind and the entity perceiving the mind. The mind cannot be a vehicle for images and, at the same time, see itself presenting them. Isn't it a shame that only our misfortunes and lack of success induce us occasionally to observe our mental faculty?

As it appears here, the mind presents objects to the spiritual entity without interruption or distortion. Interruptions are instants when one is absent, which weakens understanding. Distortions are tied up with ignorance (avidy), which is full of preconceived ideas, taboos, and so on.

ekasamaye cobhayānavadhāraṃam
ekasamaye ca-ubhaya-anavadhāraṇam

Ekasamaye: simultaneously. *Ca:* and. *Ubhaya:* of the two. *Anavadhāraṇam:* the non-grasp, incomprehension.

If consciousness of one's own consciousness originated from another state of consciousness, there would then be infinite regression of phenomena and confusion of memory.

How important is it to be lucid about the points of view that guide my behavior?

Can I do without my mind as an instrument? What happens if I spend all my time polishing up my instrument so I never have time to use it?

What disadvantage is there in using an unprepared instrument?

What can we think about the following phrase: "The mind, in effect, is the cause of both slavery and liberation" (Laws of Manu)?

This aphorism proves the teaching in aphorisms IV.19 and IV.20: the mind has no consciousness, and we cannot perceive the two levels of being simultaneously. So, to establish his demonstration, Patañjali reasons using the absurd: What would happen if the mind was aware of itself? There would then be perpetual, automatic generation of sources of consciousness. Here he refutes certain schools of thought, such as Buddhism.

A person's world influences his or her own difficulties, those of others, and one's own evolution. If I suffer from intense fear, stopping my mind will not get rid of it. The mind is unconscious, so it cannot itself create the fear I feel. Rather, fear is the result of erroneous mental function that must be purified. The negative vision must be replaced by a positive one that mirrors reality.

cittāntaradṛśye buddhibuddheratiprasaṅgaḥ smṛtisaṅkaraśca
cittāntaradṛśye buddhi-buddheḥ atiprasaṅgaḥ smṛti-saṅkaraḥ-ca

Cittāntaradṛśye: in a mind being perceived by another. *Buddhi-buddheḥ:* being conscious of one's own consciousness. *Atiprasaṅgaḥ:* plethoric manifestation. *Smṛti:* memory. *Saṅkaraḥ:* confusion. *Ca:* and.

IV.22

**When the mind is not turned outward,
it reflects consciousness itself.**

Am I extroverted? What conclusion can I draw?

What can a search for inner life bring me?

How can I attain this without neglecting my responsibilities?

What is it that sustains my interest in the outside world?

If we are neither our worries nor our peaceful states, who are we?

This aphorism points the way for those who wish to perceive the origin of consciousness in themselves. Attraction to exterior objects entails a movement of thought. Outside is what is outside the body, but also what is outside the spiritual entity: thoughts, sentiments, and emotions. A cake's smell provokes desire, the flow of saliva, and tasting—so many external elements.

Becoming aware of the external origin of thoughts is essential to realizing the state in which the mind reflects consciousness rather than objects. In this state, faced with a two-way mirror, we see our own image, or else the objects on the other side, depending on the lighted space. This spiritual experience—inwardness—in which the outside world has lost all interest, is unchanging and cannot be handed down to another.

Patañjali here refutes a possible state beyond the consituent qualities of nature that is characterless (*nirguṇa*). There is always perception of form—beyond the perception of exterior objects is perception of the form of one's own consciousness. We can list three degrees of individual consciousness (*asmitā*): suffering and pleasure (*asmitā-kleśa*); contemplation (*asmitā-samādhi*); absence of individual consciousness (*asmitā*-non-*asmitā*).

citerapratisaṅkramāyāstadākārāpattau svabhuddhisaṃvedanam
citeḥ-apratisaṅkramāyāḥ-tad-ākāra-āpattau
svabuddhi-saṃvedanam

Citeḥ: of consciousness. *Apratisaṅkramāyāḥ:* which, who feels no movement toward. *Tad-ākāra*: that form of consciousness. *Āpattau:* in the attaining. *Svabuddhi:* consciousness of self. *Saṃvedanam:* complete understanding.

Colored by the spiritual entity that perceives and by what is perceived, the mind manifests all objects.

Does my mind contribute to developing my personality? How?

When is it desirable to develop, lessen, or simply optimize the way my mind works?

Is it helpful to accept that my mind fluctuates?

Patañjali asserts that it is impossible to wipe out the mind. Is this cause for hope or despair?

Here, Patañjali presents the mind as different from both the perceiving spiritual entity and from the object perceived. He points out that it can relate to one or the other: it can perceive all. It is, therefore, constantly changing as much in its role as in its qualities. After choosing the terms *dṛṣṭar* (perceiving spiritual entity) and *dṛśya* (the perceived), Patañjali emphasizes perception. The two equivalents retained in the *Sāṃkhya* system are much more complex (*puruṣa, prakṛti*).

This aphorism presents two modes of mental functioning:

- The spiritual entity perceives the object via the mind.
- The spiritual entity perceives itself for its own illumination, via the mind.

Any other possibility is provisionally excluded, thus the spiritual entity cannot perceive the object without using the mind. This aphorism, therefore, refutes the systems that recommend reduction or suppression of the mind. It advises we clarify it and search for transparency.

dṛṣṭṛdṛśyoparaktaṃ cittaṃ sarvārtham
dṛṣṭṛ-dṛśya-uparaktaṃ cittaṃ sarva-artham

Draṣṭṛ: spiritual entity. *Dṛśya:* what is perceived or observed. *Uparaktaṃ:* colored by. *Cittam:* mind. *Sarvārtham:* totality, object, aim, meaning, etc.

IV.24

Although diversified by countless latencies, the mind exists on behalf of the higher entity associated with it.

What ways of life, activities, human relationships, leisure pursuits, and food can strengthen my mind or the priority of the spiritual entity?

Can obstacles help me to discover the superior role of the spiritual entity?

This aphorism seems to be saying, "No head, no organization." Why is it difficult to recognize the role of chief in oneself?

Is yoga a destructive or constructive process for the personality and why?

Having recalled the necessity of the mind to allow manifestation of objects, Patañjali approaches its relationship with the spiritual entity. The mind does not exist for its own sake and has only one function: to enable the spiritual entity to become aware. It is a whole life's history. The child awakens to the outer world. One day dissatisfaction appears and starts the search for an inner, higher dimension. In short, the seen universe and the mind of which it is part are necessary for freeing themselves from themselves.

The mind's numerous and varied latencies give it importance, however, there must be something in a position of responsibility—the spiritual entity. At the slightest obstacle, the mind refuses to follow the guide. To discover its presence once more, we must question ourselves: "Where is my place?" "Where do I stand?" "Who am I?"

The association of the spiritual entity and what is perceived is compared in the *Sāṃkhya-kārikā* to a blind man and a lame man lost in a forest. They can only get free by helping one another. The lame man, carried by the blind man, has to direct the other, who must follow instructions.

tadasaṅkhyeyavāsanābhiścitramapi parārthaṃ
saṃhatyakāritvāt
tad-asaṅkhyeya-vāsanābhiḥ-citram-api parārthaṃ
saṃhatya-kāritvāt

Tad: that. *Asaṅkhyeya:* innumerable. *Vāsanābhiḥ:* through latencies. *Citraṃ:* varied. *Api:* even. *Parārtham:* have the other as higher aim. *Saṃhatya-kāritvāt:* as an associated agent.

One with discerning perception is freed from all searching for the inner being.

Do I have a lot of questions about myself, others, and life in general?

If I am quiet during a meeting, is it through shyness, ignorance, respect, or wisdom?

In a one-on-one relationship, am I the one who talks the most or who listens the most?

What relationship should I draw between the quality and length of a speech and the degree of freedom of the speaker?

How do I distinguish the silence that stems from a communication problem from the silence that reflects the state described in this aphorism?

What qualities favor respect for silence?

Is it always true that the more one knows the less one says about it?

As long as the slightest wish to discover one's inner being subsists, one has not attained the state described in this aphorism. When one attains this high level of deep peace, all curiosity about going beyond it disappears. All questioning ceases and all useless words as well: the yogi falls silent, *muni.* He or she does not push forward without purpose.

We can say that the more the exceptional develops, the more speech dwindles away. It goes without saying that such silence is not the result of difficulties in relationship, quite the contrary. The wise person expresses him- or herself as much on ultimate reality as on the universe. All the great inspired texts constitute marvellous examples of communication. What comes to a stop is not the expression of life itself, but that of interrogation on the origin of life. As Vyāsa reminds us, "When a wise one talks about a deep inner dimension, the ignoramus claps and the sage weeps."

viśeṣadarśinaḥ ātmabhāvabhvanānivṛttiḥ
viśeṣa-darśinaḥ ātmabhāva-bhāvanā nivṛttiḥ

Viśeṣa: distinction, specificity. *Darśinaḥ:* of one who perceives. *Ātmabhāva:* consciousness of self. *Bhāvanā:* manifestation. *Nivṛttiḥ:* ceasing, stopping.

IV.26

The mind is then absorbed in discernment, oriented toward serenity.

Do people see me as making the right choice at the right moment? If not, what can I do about it?

Am I always in a state of inner peace and if not, how can I change that?

Can I be at once wise and clumsy?

What feeling might be at the root of a lack of involvement in active life?

If certain knowledge is to remain proprietary, how can I assure that?

How can one prepare another to receive the truth?

How can one reconcile charity or compassion and respect for another?

This aphorism further develops the concepts of discernment and serenity. First of all, the aptitude for making the right choice at the right moment is discernment that follows two obligatory requirements: reflection and action. Wisdom should translate itself into concrete facts. Would we value the knowledge of someone who says, "I know," but gives no elaboration? Discernment must be proved in active life. It is, therefore, the more important of the two directions: it is the force that pulls one toward serenity. The resulting serenity is a state of inner peace perceived as withdrawal from the whirl of life. To resume, we must accept reality and live in it without losing ourselves.

Discernment often leads one not to reply. Who is ready to know the truth about him- or herself, even if asked for? The sage is careful not to speak too quickly, to think or act for another, to overprotect.

tadā vivekanimnaṃ kaivalyaprāgbhāraṃ cittam
tadā viveka-nimnaṃ kaivalya-prāgbhāraṃ cittam

Tadā: then. *Viveka:* discernment. *Nimnam:* turned to, toward, immersed in. *Kaivalya:* independence, serenity. *Prāgbhāram:* near, turned toward. *Cittam:* the mind.

When discernment lapses, disturbing inner mental experiences rush forth due to past permeations.

Am I more in danger when everything is going well or when everything is going wrong?

What qualities can help us tolerate backsliding so we can bounce back again?

Does this aphorism imply there is never any definite victory?

What is the attitude to take when former mental states surge up again?

What connection is there between aphorism III.12 and this one?

This aphorism implies that we can never claim to have definitely overcome our difficulties. Life in all its forms shackles us. Even if it is possible and desirable to free oneself from one's bonds, extreme vigilance is needed all the while one is in the body.

Disturbing inner experiences include all speech, all behavior in judgment of others, and all egocentric thoughts such as "my" or "mine" or "I know." The more exacting we are regarding ourselves, the less we should be toward others: the higher the level of experience and responsibility we reach, the more time we should devote to preparing our speech and our actions until the end of our days, for we can no longer correct the negative effects of our latest mistakes once we die.

The kinds of mental states reactivated are manifold, the strongest being attraction to a partner. Under that heading, a couple's relationship is one of continual adjustment, whether the partners are engaged or not in a process of inner evolution.

tacchidreṣu pratyayāntarāṇi saṃskārebhyaḥ
tat-chidreṣu pratyayāntarāṇi saṃskārebhyaḥ

Tat: of this (latter) (the mind). *Chidreṣu:* in the breaking down, intervals, gaps, chinks. *Pratyayāntarāṇi:* inner mental experience. *Saṃskārebhyaḥ:* because of mental permeation.

IV.28

It is said that to abandon these states is to abandon the causes of suffering.

What causes me to lose hope?

How can I get over these setbacks?

What is the indispensable quality for beginning again?

What is the connection between this aphorism and the inability to sustain a certain level of attainment (I.30)?

What connection is there between the teaching contained in this aphorism and the notion of evolution in time, from infancy to death?

This aphorism means that we should not content ourselves with old states that the new personality has outgrown. It points out the means to be used when certain states of mind burst into activity again. The most effective is to diminish them by using simple ways that for centuries have proved their worth in eliminating causes of suffering (II.3), or other simple means adapted to recent evolution.

Even if we are tempted to believe we have "made it," we must be untiring about beginning again, unceasingly putting oureselves in question, and returning again and again to the starting point. We should not hesitate to ask for help from an experienced person once again, even if we have believed ourselves, at some time, to be able to do without it.

As we age, and decay becomes more and more difficult to slow down on the psychic and physical levels, the spiritual level itself is worth special effort, so we can avoid weakness and prepare for liberation.

hānamṣāeṣāṃ kleśavaduktam
hānam-eṣāṃ kleśavat-uktam

Hnam: abandon, loss. *Eṣām:* of these (latter). *Kleśavat:* as in the case of causes of suffering. *Uktam:* it is said, they say.

Moreover, with complete disinterest even in the higher understanding born of meditation, regardless of time, place, or circumstances, discernment brings contemplation borne on a cloud of virtuous harmony.

How can I detach myself from my successes and from my positive influence over others?

What are the signs of this state and how do others respond to it?

Can a person in this state still hesitate, make mistakes, or be influenced from outside?

If one has two roles—pupil or teacher, father or son—how might this call for different attitudes?

Just as a tropical rain cloud nourishes new life, the contemplative state described here brings with it happiness, perfection, felicity. This shower of grace can only proceed from the higher Being. If only one being attains this state, he or she nourishes generations. This state of contemplation recalls aphorism I.51. At that moment, all permeation stops. One is completely disinterested in total understanding, is beyond all doubt, whatever the circumstances.

The yogi shows knowledge, wisdom, and detachment. The more the yogi detaches from powers, the more powers are possessed and the more good is done. Such a one does not flaunt knowledge or become an unbearable mirror for another. Such a one is charisma and simplicity incarnate. He or she correctly and judiciously perceives action, its absence, and details of its execution (*Bagavad Gītā,* fourth chapter). A master, conscious that he or she is a witness and not a source, never forgets that the pupil contains all.

prasaṅkhyāne'pyakusīdasya sarvathā
vivekakhyāterdharmameghaḥ samādhiḥ
prasaṅkhyāne-api-akusīdasya sarvathā
viveka-khyāteḥ-dharma-meghaḥ samādhiḥ

Prasaṅkhyāne: higher understanding. *Api:* even, also. *Akusīdasya:* of complete disinterest. *Sarvathā:* in all ways, in any case. *Viveka:* discernment. *Khyāteḥ:* recognition. *Dharma:* order, laws. *Meghaḥ:* cloud. *Samādhiḥ:* contemplation.

IV.30

Then, on this level, all action based on afflictions has vanished.

Are my actions still based on afflictions (kleśa-s)?

Should the motives for my acts interest me?

How do we recognize when an action is based on affliction, and how can we avoid it?

If practice cannot bring us this state, can reflection and acceptance help?

What is the connection between yoga , which gives priority to direct experience, and the need to daily test one's state in action?

This aphorism presents the results of the state described in aphorism IV.29. Actions do not stop, but they are no longer born of negative attitudes (II.3)—ignorance, consciousness of I, passion, repulsion, and fear.

This new state is natural and permanent. It liberates us from all apprehension of causing something negative, for in all circumstances, action is judicious and correct. It is born of compassion—borne on the cloud of virtuous harmony.

It is the result of liberation (*kaivalya*). No practice is sufficient to attain liberation, for it is a conditioning factor. At this level, neither excessive inertia (*tamas*) nor overactivity (*rajas*) nor their inappropriate manifestations exist.

Each day, life tests this state in action. One no longer shows one's superior value, nor attachment to, nor reaction against, nor fear. Action in this state proceeds from real detachment.

tataḥ kleśakarmanivṛttiḥ
tataḥ kleśa-karma-nivṛttiḥ

Tataḥ: afterward. *Kleśa:* torments, afflictions. *Karma:* act, action. *Nivṛttiḥ:* stopping, ceasing.

Then knowledge is more or less infinite, all impurity has been repulsed, and little remains to be known.

Am I always questioning my inner state?

What is it like to ask fewer and fewer questions, yet see more and more evidence?

How can inertia, activism, or any other negative impulse (kleśa-s) mask knowledge?

When one faces an obstacle with calmness, are others likely to misunderstand this? What can one conclude from this?

Introduced by then (*tadā*) or afterwards (*tataḥ*), these last aphorisms link different facets of a unified state of being. The notion that a cloud of impurities hides omniscience recalls that each being potentially bears knowledge and wisdom within. The meaning of "impurity" (*mala*) includes toxins, as well as wrong thoughts or attitudes. Such impurities disappear when knowledge becomes practically infinite.

Here knowledge is concrete. It concerns what we can perceive, learn, and communicate. We then reach the limits of what we can learn. This wisdom shows itself, in particular, when we face obstacles associated with the five causes of affliction and exterior events. Everything that would have been a major obstacle before, now has no gravity. Problems are seen in their correct proportions. They are neither insoluble nor serious.

Still, however, we must remain vigilant, for no knowledge is perfect. In fact, the more we know, the more we are conscious of the immense amount that remains to be explored. At this high level of self-knowledge, learning is nothing. If life demands new knowledge, apprenticeship will be easy.

tadā sarvāvaraṇamalāpetasya jñānasyānantyājjñeyamalpam
tad sarva-varaa-mala-apetasya jñānasya-nantyt-jeyam-alpam

Tadā: then. *Sarva:* all, everywhere. *Āvaraṇa:* that which covers, masks. *Mala:* impurity. *Apetasya:* lacking in, deprived of, repulsed, pushed away. *Jñānasya:* of knowledge. *Ānantyāt:* because of the ultimate, extreme limit. *Jñeyam:* to be known. *Alpam:* little.

IV.32

Then, for the constituent qualities of nature, their end is accomplished and their unfolding ceases.

Am I inactive in action and active in inaction?

If I no longer hesitate, does every question give rise to a spontaneous reply that is always judicious and correct?

How can I keep from confusing indifference with the wisdom described here?

What is the connection between equanimity and this wisdom?

What is the connection between suffering and this wisdom?

For a believer, what does this wisdom correspond to?

With attainment of the state described in aphorism IV.27, inferior states could reappear because the constituent qualities of nature could still give birth to the complementarity of enjoyment and recoil (*bhoga-apavarga, II.18*). With attainment of the state introduced in this aphorism, however, the negative no longer appears from inside. Action is free of all unfavorable conditioning. One still evolves, of course, but no longer hesitates or vascillates.

A human being in this state never loses presence of mind, most noticeably in the midst of problems, when things are very challenging. For one such as this, past stages of evolution, as a whole, no longer create problems, nor do present or future transformations.

tataḥ kṛtārthānāṃ pariṇāmakramasamāptirguṇānām
tataḥ kṛta-arthānāṃ pariṇāma-krama-samāptiḥ-guṇānām

Tataḥ: then. *Kṛta:* action done, accomplished. *Arthānā:* of the aims or intent. *Pariṇāma:* changes, evolution. *Krama:* unfolding, flow, succession. *Samāptiḥ:* stopping, ceasing. *Guṇānām:* of the three constituent qualities of nature.

The succession of moments appears in the grasp of past and future changes correlative to the next moment.

Am I always chasing time?

If so, where and how can I find happiness?

How can I control my timing so I know when to wait and when to act quickly?

What is life like when perceived in the eternal present?

How does it affect me to perceive time, space, and phenomena with increasing relativity?

Can we establish a connection between the traditional Hindu view, in which both time and the universe are cyclic and there is little interest in dating historic events, and Western concepts of evolution and the need for precise, historical references?

This aphorism presents the relativity of time and relativity in general. It defines *krama,* which we translate as succession, and which corresponds to a transitory state of something evolving. This definition is based on the notion of the moment (*kṣana*), or the smallest unit of psychological time, which materializes when one becomes aware that one state has been replaced by another. Thus, time is seen only through grasping a change in at least one characteristic—the hand is not long in the same spot on the dial, I just blinked my eyelids, my mood is different, the flower has opened.

The perception of time as fluctuating is linked to several factors: the quantity of changes seen and one's appreciation of them. An unbearable meeting of a few minutes can seem like hours, while during agreeable moments, time flies.

We can perceive the phenomenal universe only through its constituent qualities (*guṇa-s*) and their never-ending changes (*paniṇāma*). When the mind steadies itself and steps back, time and other natural phenomena become relative. We become conscious of living "here and now" in an eternal present.

In a cyclic representation of time, life is seen as a wheel turning. At this high level, one is no longer on the wheel afflicted by centrifugal force—one is at the hub and contemplates time turning around him or her. One grasps the relativity of time and remains unaffected. The acute observation one has acquired allows him or her to perceive reciprocity in human relationships and thereafter favorably influence evolution.

kṣaṇapratiyogī pariṇāmāparāntanirgrāhyaḥ kramaḥ
kṣaṇa-pratiyogī pariṇāma-apara-anta-nirgrāhyaḥ kramaḥ

Kṣaṇa: instant, moment. *Pratiyogī:* correlative, face to face. *Pariṇāma:* change, evolution. *Apara:* anterior. *Anta:* posterior. *Nirgrāhyaḥ:* understanding, grasp. *Kramaḥ:* unwinding, unfolding, succession, sequence.

In liberation, the play of the constituent qualities of nature is no longer a source of meaning or interest to the spiritual entity; or, liberation is the supreme power of pure consciousness founded on itself. End.

Is my individuality only a means of self-liberation?

How can one avoid intellectualizing the steps taken and ending up in an "ivory tower"?

Will my future actions spring only from others' needs?

How can I recognize this state in another?

How can I preserve this state when being congratulated for being in it?

What makes Patañjali's treatise universal?

Patañjali brings his treatise on yoga to an end here by defining spiritual liberation. It is, first of all, defined with regard to the constituent qualities of nature, whose play and interaction have hitherto directed all of ones physical and mental activities. With liberation, this play stops and the mind no longer reacts. Though action continues, it takes place in beatitude.

Lastly, liberaton is presented with regard to pure consciousness, whose triple power shows itself: to know, to awake, to understand.

Thus Patañjali's treatise ends with the choice between two definitions of real freedom. As T. K.V. Desikachar writes: "The mind is a faithful servant to the master, the Perceiver."

puruṣārthaśūnyāṇāṃ guṇānāṃ pratiprasavaḥ kaivalyaṃ svarūpapratiṣṭhā vā citiśaktiriti

puruṣa-artha-śūnyānāṃ guṇānāṃ pratiprasavaḥ kaivalyaṃ svarūpa-pratiṣṭhā vā citiśaktiḥ-iti

Puruṣa: spiritual entity. *Artha:* aim or intent. *Śūnyānāṃ:* deprived of, lacking in, absence of. *Guṇānāṃ:* constituent qualities of nature. *Pratiprasavaḥ:* opposite, opposing production. *Kaivalyaṃ:* liberation, beatitude. *Svarūpa:* its own form, shape, its true nature. *Pratiṣṭhā:* founded on. *Vā:* or else by. *Citiśaktiḥ:* the powers of pure consciousness. *Iti:* end, here ends.

GLOSSARY

Sanskrit words are presented in this glossary depending on the following criteria:

- They are given without declensions, that is, in theme form, which explains changes in word endings;
- The alphabetical order used in the English, including Sanskrit letters with accents (diacritic signs) or else double English characters is: *a, ā, ai, au, b, c, ch, d, ḍ, dh, ḍh, e, g, gh, h, i, ī, j, jh, k, kh, l, ḷ, m, ṃ, n, ṅ, ñ, ṇ, o, p, ph, r, ṛ, ś, ṣ, s, t, ṭ, th, ṭh, u, v, y;*
- Anything relevant to the demonstrative form *tad* (*teṣam, saḥ, tasmin*) is regrouped under *tad*;
- In the same way, anything to do with the verb to be (*asti, syāt, sant, sati,* etc.) is regrouped under its indicative *as.*

A

A (an): negative prefix; cf. for example *hiṃsā* II.23 and *a-hiṃsā* II.30
Abhāva: absence I.10, 29, II.25, IV.11
Abhibhava: suppression III.9
Abhijāta: purified I.41
Abhimata: wished for I.39
Abhiniveśa: fear II.3, 9
Abhivyakti: manifestation IV.8
Abhyāsa: persevering practice I.12, 13, 18, 32
Adṛṣṭa: not seen II.12
Adhigama: obtaining I.29
Adhimātrā: strong I.22, II.34
Adhiṣṭhātṛtva: supremacy III.49
Adhva-bheda: different moments IV.12
Adhyāsa: false attribution III.17
Adhyātman: Supreme Being I.47
Ahiṃsā: nonviolence II.30, 35
Ajñāna: ignorance II.34
Ajñāta: unknown IV.17
Akalpita: not conceived, unconceived III.43
Akaraṇa: avoiding III.51
Akliṣṭa: not producing suffering I.5
Akṛṣṇa: not somber IV.7
Akrama: without taking steps III.54
Akusīda: complete desinterest IV.29
Alabdha-bhūmikatva: incapacity to attain a new stage I.30
Aliṅga: absence of distinctive marking I.45, II.19
Alpa: little IV.31
Aṅga: member, limb II.28, 29, 40, III.7, 8
Aṅgam-ejayatva: physical agitation I.31
Añjanatā: characteristics I.41
Aṇiman: miniaturization III.45
Anabhighāta: invulnerability II.48, III.45

Ananta: the infinite, infinity II.34, 47,
Anaṣṭaṃ: not destroyed, still appearing II.22,
Anavaccheda: not to be limited I.26, III.53
Anavacchinna: not limited by II.31
Anavadhāraṇa: not grasped IV.20
Anavasthitatva: the impossibility of remaining at the level reached I.30
Anāditva: without origin IV.10
Anāgata: has not yet happened or occurred II.16, III.16, IV.12
Anāśaya: absence of latencies IV.6
Anātman: nonabsolute II.5,
Aneka: many others IV.5
Aniṣṭa: undesirable III.51
Anitya: temporary II.5
Anta: posterior, limit I.40, IV.33
Antar-aṅga: internal member III.7
Antara: interior IV.2
Antarāya: obstacle I.29,I.30
Antardhāna: disappearance III.21
Anvaya: as far as ... is concerned III.9
Anubhūta: experimented, experienced I.11
Anugama: following on (which) I.17
Anuguṇa: appropriate IV.8
Anukāra: resemblance, likeness II.54
Anumāna: inference I.7,I.49
Anumodita: approved II.34
Anupaśya: continually perceived II.20
Anupātin: formed of I.9, III.14
Anuśayin: that which follows II.7, II.8
Anuśāsana: exposition, statement (of facts) I.1
Anuṣṭhāna: execution, carry out II.28
Anuttama: highest II.42
Anvaya: relation, relationship III.44, 47
Anya: other I.18, 49, 50, II.22
Anyatā: difference III.49, 53
Anyatva: is different III.15
Apara: anterior IV.33
Aparāmṛṣṭa: not attained by I.24
Aparānta: final ending III.22
Aparigraha: noncovetousness II.30, 39
Apariṇāmitva: unevolving state IV.18
Apavarga: liberation, freedom II.18
Apekṣitva: the gaze on IV.17
Apeta: lacking (not provided with) IV.31
Api: also, even, same I.22, 26, 29, 51, II.20, 22, III.8, 50, IV.9, 24, 29
Apramāṇaka: that which is only IV.16
Apratisaṅkrama: which feels no movement toward IV.22
Aprayojaka: inoperative IV.3
Apuṇya: vice, incorrect I.33, II.14
Ariṣṭa: portent, omen III.22
Artha: meaning, essence, aim, intent I.28, 32, 42, 43, 49, II.2, 18, 21, 22, III.3, 17, IV.32, 34
Arthavattva: value based on the goal III.44, 47
Aśuci: impure, unclean II.5
Aśuddhi: impurity, uncleanness II.28, 43
Aśukla: not luminous IV.7
Aṣṭa: eight II.29
As: to be IV.12, 16
Asaṃpramoṣa: retention I.11
Asaṃprayoga: separation II.54, III.21
Asaṃsarga: no contact II.40
Asaṅga: not affected III.39
Asaṅkīra: distinct III.35
Asaṅkhyeya: innumerable IV.24
Asmitā: consciousness of I, the ego I.17, II.3, 6, III.47, IV.4

Asteya: not stealing II.30, 37
Asti: see *As*
Asya: see *Tad*
Atadrūpa: a form different from what it is I.8
Atiprasaṅga: plethoric manifestation IV.21
Atīta: the past III.16, IV.12
Atha: and now, this is I.1
Atyanta: beyond all limits III.35
Avasthā: situation III.13
Avasthāna: establishment, set up I.3,
Avidyā: misconception, misrecognition II.3, 4, 5, 24
Aviplava: total clarity II.26
Avirati: intemperance I.30
Aviṣayin: without object, objectless III.20
Aviśeṣa: nonspecific II.19, III.35
Avyapadeśya: the future III.14

Ā

Ā: until, up to II.28
Ābhyantara: internal II.50, II.51
Ādara: respect I.14
Ādarśa: clairvoyance III.36
Ādi: the beginning, etc. II.34, III.23, 24, 39, 45
Āgamā: faithful testimony, revelation I.7
Ākāśa: ether, space III.41, 42
Ākṣepin: complete rejection, going beyond II.51
Ālambana: support, base I.10, 38, IV.11
Ālasya: apathy I.30
Āloka: sparkle, brilliance III.25
Ānanda: beatitude I.17,
Ānantarya: continuity IV.9
Ānantya: ultimate limit IV.31
Ānuśravika: heard, tradition I.15
Āpatti: attainment. IV.22
Āpūra: pouring IV.2
Āsana: posture II.29, 46
Āsanna: near I.21
Āśaya: latent impression I.24, II.12
Āsevita: nourished, fed by I.14,
Āśis: life instinct, possession instinct IV.10
Āśraya: mental coloring IV.11
Āśrayatva: a close relationship exists II.36
Āsvāda: refined taste III.36
Ātman: Absolute, essence II.5, 21, 41, IV.13, 18, 25
Ātmabhāva: consciousness of self IV.25
Ātmaka: considering in II.18, IV.13, 18, 25
Ātmatā: principle II.6
Āvaraṇa: veil II.52, III.43, IV.31
Āveśa: taking possession III.38
Āyus: longevity II.13

B

Bahis: exterior, external III.8, 43
Bala: force III.23, 24, 46
Bandha: link III.1, 38
Bādhana: harassment II.33
Bāhya: external II.50, 51
Bīja: seed I.25, III.50
Brahmacarya: continence II.30, 38
Buddhi-buddhi: aware of one's own consciousness IV.21

BH

Bhara: bearer of I.48
Bhauma: earth II.31
Bhāva: existing, state I.19, III.48
Bhāvana: manifestation I.28, I.33, II.2, 33, 34, IV.25
Bheda: piercing, fragmentation IV.3, 5, 15
Bhoga: enjoyment, experience II.13, 18, III.35
Bhrāntidarśana: error of judgment I.30
Bhūmi: ground I.14, III.6
Bhūta: the five gross elements (ether, air, fire, water, earth), creature II.18, III.13, 17, 20, 44

Bhuvana: world III.26

C

Ca: and I.29, 44, 45, II.2, 15, 41, 53, III.20, 22, 38, 39, 42, 45, 48, 49, 54, IV.10, 16, 20, 21
Cakṣus: eye III.21
Cakra: energy center of the body III.29
Candra: moon III.27
Caturtha: fourth II.51
Cet: if IV.16
Cetana: consciousness I.29
Citi: consciousness IV.22
Citiśakti: powers of pure consciousness IV.34
Citra: varied IV.24
Citta: psyche, spirit, mind I.2, 30, 33, 37, II.54, III.1, 9, 11, 12, 19, 34, 38, IV.4, 5, 15, 16, 17, 18, 23, 26
Cittāntaradṛśya: a mind in the process of being seen by another IV.21

CH

Chidra: rupture, break IV.27

D

Darśana: vision, point of view, doctrine I.30, II.6, 41, III.32
Darśin: one who perceives IV.25
Daurmana: nervous breakdown I.31
Deśa: space II.31, 50, III.1, 53, IV.9
Devatā: divinity II.44
Dīpti: light, brilliance II.28
Dīrgha: long I.14, II.50,
Divya: divine III.41
Doṣa: blemish, humor, impurity III.50
Draṣṭar: the perceiving, observing entity I.3, II.17, 20, IV.23
Dṛḍha: firm I.14
Dṛg: one who perceives II.6
Dṛśi: vision II.25
Dṛśimātra: vision only II.20
Dṛṣṭa: seen, visible universe I.15, II.12
Dṛśya: the perceived, object II.17, 18, 21 IV.23
Dṛśyatva: being perceived IV.19
Duḥkha: pain I.31, 33, II.5, 8, 15, 16, 34
Dvandva: opposing pairs II.48
Dveṣa: aversion II.3, 8

DH

Dharma: law, order III.13, 14, 45, IV.12, 29
Dharmin: fundamental characteristic III.14
Dhāraṇā: concentration II.29, 53, III.1
Dhruva: Pole Star, immutable III.28
Dhyāna: meditation I.39, II.11, 29, III.2, IV.6

E

Eka: one I.32, II.6, IV.5, 16
Ekarūpatva: similarity IV.9
Ekatānatā: fixed a long while on one point III.2
Ekatra: on one point III.4
Ekatva: unity IV.14
Ekasamaye: simultaneouly IV.20
Ekāgratā: focusing III.11, 12
Ekāgrya: orientation on one point II.41
Eṣa: this I.44, III.13, IV.11, 28
Eva: precisely I.44, 46, II.15, 21, III.3, IV.8

G

Gamana: displacement, crossing III.42
Gati: movement II.49, III.28
Grahaṇa: instrument of perception I.41, III.47
Grahītar: perceiving agent I.41
Grāhya: perceived object I.41, III.21

Guṇa: constituent qualities of nature I.16, II.15, 19, IV.13, 32, 34
Guru: master, guide I.26

H

Hastin: elephant III.24
Hāna: cessation II.25, 26, IV.28
Heya: what must be avoided II.10, 11, 16, 17
Hetu: cause II.17, 23, 24, III.15, IV.11
Hetutva: is a cause II.14
Hiṃsā: does harm, evil II.34
Hlāda: joy II.14
Hṛdaya: heart III.34

I

Indriya: organs of perception, action, and thought II.18, 41, 43, 54, 55, III.13, 47
Iṣṭa: desired, chosen II.44
Itaratra: otherwise, elsewhere I.4
Itara: others I.20, IV.7
Itaretara: one and another, mutual III.17
Iti: end, such is II.34, III.54, IV.34
Iva: as if, so to say I.41, 43, II.6, 54, III.3

Ī

Īśvara: God, Lord I.23, 24
Īśvara-praṇidhāna: devotion to the Lord II.1, 32, 45

J

Ja: born of I.50, III.52, 54, IV.1, 6
Jala: water. III.39
Janma: birth, origin II.12, II.39, IV.1
Japa: repetition I.28
Javitva: promptness, instantaneousness III.48
Jaya: victory II.41, III.5, 39, 40, 44, 47, 48
Jāti: caste, rank II.13, 31, III.18, 53, IV.2, 9
Jāyante: are produced, appear III.36
Jñāna: knowledge I.8, 9, 38, 42, II.28, III.16, 17, 18, 19, 22, 25, 26, 27, 28, 29, 35, 52, 54, IV.31
Jñāta: perceived, known IV.17, 18
Jñeyam: to be known IV.31
Jugupsā: care, keeping II.40
Jvalana: radiance III.40
Jyotis: light III.32
Jyotiṣmatī: luminous I.36

K

Kaivalya: liberation, serenity II.25, III.50, 55, IV.26, 34
Kāla: time, time span I.14, 26, II.31, 50, IV.9
Kaṇṭaka: thorns III.39
Kaṇṭha: throat, neck III.30
Karaṇa: production, act II.2
Karman: action, act I.24, II.12, III.22, IV.7, 30
Karuṇā: compassion, pity I.33
Kathaṃtā: reason II.39
Kāraṇa: cause, origin III.38
Kārita: caused, occasioned, provoked II.34
Kāya: body II.43, III.21, 29, 42, 45, 46
Kiṃ: is...? How? IV.16
Kleśa: cause of suffering, affliction I.24, II.2, 3, 12, IV.30
Kleśavat: as for causes of suffering IV.28
Kliṣṭa: productive of suffering, painful I.5
Krama: progression, succession III.15, 52, IV.32, 33
Kriyā: action, religious act II.1, 18, 36
Krodha: anger, fury II.34
Kṛta: realized, accomplished II.22, 34, IV.32
Kṣaṇa: instant, smallest unit of time III.9, 52, IV.33
Kṣaya: destruction, elimination II.28, 43, III.11, 43, 50

Kṣetra: terrain, ground, field II.4
Kṣetrikavat: like a gardener IV.3
Kṣīṇa: diminished, reduced I.41
Kṣīyate: is destroyed, reduced II.52
Kṣudh: hunger III.30
Kūpa: cavity, hole III.30
Kūrma: toirtoise, earth considered as a tortoise; second reincarnation of Viṣṇu, one of the ten breaths (*prāṇa*) III.31

KH

Khyāti: become aware of I.16, II.5, 26, 28, III.49, IV.29

L

Lakṣaṇa: time, period III.13, 53
Laghu: light, rapid III.42
Lābha: obtaining, gain II.38, 42
Lāvaṇya: attractiveness, charm III.46
Liṅgamātra: differentiated, difference II.19
Lobha: avidity, haste II.34
Loka: light III.5

M

Madhya: medium, intermediary I.22, II.34
Mahā: great II.31
Mahattva: greatness I.40
Mahāvideha: superior, higher state where one is freed from the body III.43
Maitrī: friendship, love I.33, III.23
Mala: impurity IV.31
Manas: thought I.35, II.53, III.48
Mani: precious stone, jewel, gem I.41
Mantra: sacred formula or word IV.1
Mātra: (when ending a word), only, nothing but I.43, III.3, 49, IV.4
Megha: cloud IV.29
Mithyā: incorrect, false I.8
Moha: mental aberration II.34
Mṛdu: soft, tender, slow I.22, II.34
Muditā: joy I.33
Mūla: root, foundation, origin II.12, 13
Mūrdhan: top of the head III.32

N

Na: no, non, not III.20, IV.16, 19
Nairantarya: without interruption, continuity I.14
Naṣṭa: disappeared, vanished, destroyed II.22
Nābhi: navel, umbilicus III.29
Nāḍī: canal, artery, tubular organ, pulse III.31
Nibandhinī: linked, bound, which links, binds I.35
Nidrā: deep sleep (dreamles)I.6, 10, 38,
Nimna: turned toward, immersed in IV.26
Niratiśaya: unsurpassed, unequalled I.25
Nirbhāsa: manifestation, appearance, brilliance I.43, III.3
Nirbīja: (contemplation) without seed I.51, III.8
Nimitta: cause, reason IV.3
Nirgrāhyā: understanding, grasp IV.33
Nirmāṇa: measure, influence IV.4
Nirodha: stoppage, control I.2, 12, 51, III.9
Nirupakrama: slow evolution III.22
Nirvicāra: subtle contemplation I.44, 47
Nirvitarka: contemplation beyond analytical knowledge I.43
Nitya: eternal, permanent II.5
Nityatva: eternal character, permanent IV.10
Nivṛtti: stopping, ceasing IV.25, 30
Niyama: attitudes toward oneself II.29, 32

Nyāsa: put down, abandon, renunciation III.25

O

Oṣadhi: consecrated plants during a ritual IV.1

P

Paṅka: mud III.39

Pañcatayya: of five kinds I.5

Panthan: path, way IV.15

Para: other, different, ultimate extreme, supreme I.16, II.40, III.19, 38

Parama: supreme, the extreme I.40, II.55

Paramāṇu: infinitely small, infinitesimal part I.40

Parārtha: take another as higher aim IV.24

Parārthatva: because of another aim, goal III.35

Paridṛṣṭa: observed, mastered II.50,

Pariṇāma: transformation or change due to time, mutation II 15, III.11, 12, 13, 15, 16, IV.2, 14, 32, 33

Pariśuddhi: complete purification I.43

Paritāpa: burn, anguish, repentance II.14

Parvan: stage,degree, division II.19

Paryavasānam: at its end, ending up at I.45

Pāda: chapter, foot, quarter I, II, III, IV

Pipāsā: thirst III.30

Prabhū: master, lord IV.18

Pracāra: movement III.38

Pracchardana: breathing out, exhale I.34

Pradhāna: first cause, origin III.48

Prajñā: highest knowledge, wisdom I.20, 48, 49, II.27, III.5

Prakāśa: light, apparition II.18, 52, III.21, 43

Prakṛti: nature, matter IV.2, 13

Prakṛtilaya: beings reabsorbed in original matter I.19

Pramāda: effervescence, lack of concentration I.30

Pramāṇa: correct mental grasp, well-founded grasp I.6, 7

Praṇava: the Sacred Syllable I.27

Prāṇāyāma: breathing exercises, breath control II.29, 49

Praṇidhāna: active devotion I.23

Prasāda: serenity, clarity, illumination I.47,

Prasādana: purification, serenity, tranquillity I.33

Prasaṅga: bad inclination, leanings, harmful inclination III.51

Prasaṅkhyāna: total and higher grasp, fruit of meditation IV.29

Praśānta: appeased III.10

Prasupta: asleep, latent II.4

Praśvāsa: irregular, unharmonious breathing II.49

Prati: regarding II.22

Pratibandhin: opposes I.50

Pratipakṣa: opposite side, opposite part II.33, 34,

Pratipatti: discriminative knowledge, distinction III.53

Pratiprasava: ceases production, inverse movement IV.34

Pratiṣedha: elimination, control I.32

Pratiṣṭha: foundation, stability I.8, II.35, 36, 37, 38, IV.34

Pratyāhāra: withdrawal of the senses from objects II.29, 54

Pratyak: turned inwards I.29

Pratyaka: sensory perception I.7

Prayatnṣa: correct, judicious, appropriate effort II.47

Pratyaya: mental experience, contents of mind I.10, 18, 19, II.20, III.2, 12, 17, 19, 35

Pratyayāntara: inner mental experience IV.27

Samārūḍha: that which has developed, that which has firmly established itself II.9
Samaya: circumstances II.31
Saṃbandha: about relation III.41, 42
Saṃbodhaḥ: total knowledge, deep understanding II.39
Saṃhananatva: firmness, solidness, solidity, endurance III.46
Saṃhatya-kāritva: in the quality of associated agent IV.24
Saṃjñā: consciousness, becoming perfectly aware, conscious I.15
Saṃkhyā: number, count, name of a system of thought II.50
Saṃpad: plenitude, fullness, blooming III.45, 46
Saṃprajñāta: contemplation with cognitive consciousness of an object I.17
Saṃprayoga: union, fusion II.44
Saṃśaya: doubt, evasiveness I.30
Saṃskāra: mental permeation resulting from past acts I.18, 50, II.15, III.9, 10, 18, IV.9, 27
Saṃtoṣa: contentedness, contentment II.32, 42
Saṃvedana: complete understanding IV.22
Saṃvega: impulse, vehemence I.21
Saṃvid: complete knowledge, understanding III.34
Saṃyama: perfect mastery, renunciation III.4, 16, 17, 21, 22, 26, 35, 41, 42, 44, 47, 52
Saṃyoga: union, confusion, (mix-up), conjunction II.17, 23, 25
Saṅga: attachment, pleasure III.51
Saṅgṛhītatva: depending on the grasp IV.11
Saṅkara: confusion, mixture III.17, IV.21
Saṅkīrṇa: mixed, composed of I.42
Saṅnidha: proximity, presence II.35
Saptadhā: comprising seven parts, sevenfold II.27
Sarva: all I.51, II.15, 37, III.17, 33, IV.31
Sarvajña: omniscience I.25
Sarvabhāva: complete state of III.49
Sarvajñātṛtva: omniscience III.49
Sarvathā: in all sorts of ways, by all means, all sorts of means III.54, IV.29
Sarvathāviṣaya: for any form of object, at any level III.54
Sarvārtha: the object's totality, the complete aim, goal IV.23
Sarvārthatā: multidirectional, multiplicity of objects III.11
Sant: being (see as) II.13, 49
Satkāra: seriousness, rectitude I.14
Sattva: understanding, clarity, equilibrium I.16, II.41, III.35, 49, 55
Satya: veracity, truth II.30, 36
Saumana: feeling of well-being, good humor II.41
Saṃvedana: subtle perception III.38
Savicāra: contemplation with subtle grasp, correct, judicious intuition I.44
Savitarka: with analytical knowledge, deductive I.42
Sādhāraṇatva: have in common II.22
Sākṣātkaraṇa: before one's eyes, perception III.18
Sālambanam: with support III.20
Sāmya: identical, equal III.55, IV.15
Sārūpya: identification I.4
Siddha: realized being, success III.32, 37, IV.1
Siddhi: power, perfection II.43, 45
Smaya: marveling, astonishment III.51
Smṛti: memory I.6, 11, 20, 43, IV.9, 21

Sopakrama: with evolution or rapid steps III.22
Stambha: suspension, suppression II.50, III.21
Sthairya: firmness, stability, calm II.39, III.31
Sthānin: superior, higher being, elevated position III.51
Sthira: firm, stable, worthy of confidence, established II.46
Sthiti: stability I.13, 35, II.18
Sthūla: gross, material, physical III.44
Styāna: inertia, mental heaviness, languor I.30
Sukha: easy, agreeable, pleasure, happiness I.33, II.5, 7, 42, 46
Sūkṣma: subtle, causal I.44, 45, II.10, 50, III.25, 44, IV.13
Śūnya: lacking in, deprived of IV.34
Sūrya: the sun III.26
Sūtra: treatise made up of aphorisms, aphorism, cord, thread.
Sva: one's own, belonging to oneself II.9, 23, 40, 54
Svabuddhi: consciousness of self IV.22
Svapna: dreaming, the dream I.38
Svarūpa: its, one's own shape, form I.3, 43, II.23, 54, III.3, 44, 47, IV.34
Svarūpata: one's own essential form IV.12
Svābhāsa: one's own essential brilliance, shine IV.19
Svādhyāya: reflection on oneself, study of sacred texts, chanting II.1, 32, 44
Svāmi: the master II.23
Svārtha: interest in the Inner Being III.35
Syāt: see as: to be

T

Tad: this one, this, that I.12, 16, 27, 28, 30, 32, 41, 46, 50, 51, II.10, 11, 13, 14, 21, 22, 24, 25, 27, 35, 49, III.3, 5, 6, 8, 10, 17, 20, 21, 22, 28, 37, 45, 50, 52, IV.8, 10, 11, 13, 15, 16, 17, 18, 19, 24, 27
Tadā: then, afterwards I.3, IV.16, 26, 31
Tad-ākāra: that form (of consciousness) IV.22
Tad-añjanatā: assuming its characteristics I.41
Tamas: inertia, incomprehension, unconsciousness I.10, 16
Tantra: depending on. IV.16
Tanu: slight, feeble, light II.2, 4
Tapas: heat, fervor, ascetic discipline, penitence II.1, II.32, 43, IV.1
Tasmin: see *Tad*
Tasya: see *Tad*
Tat: see *Tad*
Tatas: then, following l to I.22, 29, II.48, 52, 55, III.12, 36, 43, 45, 48, 53, IV.3, 8, 30, 32
Tatra: there, in that case I.13, 25, 42, 48, III.2, IV.6
Tatstha: established in that I.41
Tattva: essential principle, true nature, essence I.32, IV.14
Tayos: see *Tad*
Tāpa: burn, burning, sorrow, case II.15
Tārā: star III.27
Tārakam: transcendental, liberating, spontaneous III.54
Tāsām: see *Tad*
Tīvra: intense, ardent I.21
Te: see *Tad*
Traya: triad, three, threefold III.4, 7, 16
Trividha: of three kinds IV.7
Tu: but, however I.14, IV.3
Tulya: identical, similar III.12, 53

Tūla: cotton III.42
Tyāga: abandonment, disappearance II.35

U

Ubhaya: two IV.20
Udāna: one of the five breaths, elevating vital energy III.39
Udāra: active, abundant, manifested II.4
Udaya: emergence, appearance, apparition III.11
Udita: present, manifestation III.12, 14
Ukta: it is said IV.28
Upalabdhi: acquisition, understanding II.23
Upanimantraṇa: respectfully invited III.51
Uparāga: influence, attraction, coloring IV.17
Uparakta: colored by IV.23
Upasarga: obstacle, misfortune, unhappiness III.37
Upasthāna: approaching, of appearing II.37
Upāya: means, method, way II.26
Upekṣa: neutrality, indifference I.33
Utkrānti: ascension. III.39
Utpanna: produced by I.35
Uttara: following, next, future II.4

V

Vaira: animosity, hostility, discord, hate II.35
Vairgāya: nonattachment I.12, 15, III.50
Vaiśāradya: maturity, expert in I.47
Vaitṛṣṇya: absence of desire I.16
Vajra: diamond, thunderbolt III.46
Varaṇa: dyke, rampart IV.3
Vaśīkāra: mastery, submission to the will I.15, 40
Vastu: object, reality I.9, IV.14, 15, 16, 17
Vaśyatā: mastery II.55
Vā: or else I.23, 34, 35, 36, 37, 38, 39, III.22, 33, IV.34
Vācaka: which means, expresses, designates I.27
Vāhin: which carries, bears, transports II.9
Vāhitā: flow (wave), current, flowing away III.10
Vārta: subtle sense of smell III.36
Vāsanā: latency IV.8, 24
Vedana: subtle sense of touch III.36
Vedanīya: experimented, experienced, discovered II.12
Vibhakta: distinction, divergence IV.15
Vibhūti: accomplishment, power III
Vicāra: subtle grasp, intuitive, reflection I.17
Viccheda: stopping, interruption II.49
Vicchinna: intermittent, interrupted II.4
Videha: bodily, disincarnate I.19
Vidhāraṇa: stopping, holding, apnea, control I.34
Vidvāms: wiseman, sage, he who has knowledge II.9
Vikalpa: imagination, ideation I.6, 9, 42
Vikaraṇa: independence of the sense organs III.48
Vikṣepa: dispersion, distraction I.30, 31
Viniyoga: using, applying III.6
Vipāka: result, fruit, consequence I.24, II.13, IV.8
Viparyaya: error I.6, 8
Viprakṛṣṭa: far off, distant III.25
Virāma: halting, stopping, renouncing I.18
Virodha: contradictory character, incompatibility II.15
Vīrya: courage, energy I.20, II.38

Viṣaya: object of sensorial experience I.11, 15, 33, 37, 44, 49, II.51, 54, III.54
Viṣayatva: is an object I.45
Viṣayavant: highly objective perception I.35
Viśeṣa: specificity, specific, superior I.22, 24, 49, II.19, IV.25
Viśoka: serenity, absence of pain I.3
Vītarāga: "all passion spent," with passions appeased I.37
Vitarka: reasoning, supposition I.17, II.33, 34
Vitṛṣṇa: absence of desire I.15
Viveka: discernment, distinction II.26, 28, III.52, 54, IV.26, 29
Vivekin: one who possesses discernment, the sage II.15
Vrata: rule, observance, vow II.31
Vṛtti: psychic, mental activity I.2, 4, 5, 10, 41, II.11, 15, 50, III.43, IV.18
Vyakta: manifested, of effects IV.13
Vyavahita: out of sight, of habit, separate III.25, IV.9
Vyādhi: illness, indisposition I.30
Vyākhyātā: explained, commented I.44, III.13
Vyūha: disposal, arrangement III.27, 29
Vyutthāna: fluctuating state, activity III.9, 37

Y

Yama: attitudes toward others II.29, 30
Yathā: depending on, conforming with I.39
Yatna: tenacious, dogged effort I.13
Yoga: yogaI.1, 2, II.28
Yogin: yogi IV.7
Yogyata: aptitude, aptness II.53
Yogyatva: aptitude, aptness II.41

BIBLIOGRAPHY

Patañjali's Yoga Sūtras, Rāma Prasāda. Munshiram Manoharlal. Allahabad, 1963.

Yoga Philosophy of Patañjali, Swāmi Hariharānanda Āranya. University of Calcutta, 1963.

Yogasūtra of Patañjali, Bangali Baba. Motilal Banarsidass. Delhi, 1976.

Yogasūtra Workbook, Krisnamacharya Yoga Mandiram. Madras, 1980.

Yogasūtras of Patañjali, text with chant notation in Sanskrit and Roman script. Krisnamacharya Yoga Mandiram. Madras, 1985.

Yoga-sūtra De Patañjali, T. K. V. Desikachar. Éd. du Rocher. Paris, 1986.

Yoga-sūtras Patañjali, Françoise Mazet. Albin Michel. Paris, 1991.

ACKNOWLEDGMENTS

I wish to express my deep gratitude to my teacher and my guide on the path of yoga, T. K.V. Desikachar. The teaching contained in this book stems directly from the lessons he was good enough to give me in Madras for several years. This was personal teaching adapted for me. I hope I have been able to respect the universal application of its message.

My heartfelt thanks go to all those many other teachers of yoga, pupils, and friends—to mention a few, Jean-Pierre Jossua, Vasundhara Filliozat, Jean Varenne—who have greatly helped and encouraged me. Impossible to quote them all.

Without Corinne Abouly, Anne Bernard-Maugiron, Eveline Corominas, Franoise Devaux, Thierry Jumeau, Claudette Lefévre, Christine Lepeu, François Marméche, Béatrice Martin, Jean-Paul Martin, Michel Mercadié, André Nachin, Nicole Ponce and René Racapé, this project would never have seen light. To them my sincere thanks.

I also thank all those who can help improve the quality of this work by their remarks and suggestions.